Osteoporosis Overview - Importance of Screening and Treatment

Edited by Hechmi Toumi

Published in London, United Kingdom

Osteoporosis Overview - Importance of Screening and Treatment
http://dx.doi.org/10.5772/intechopen.1008027
Edited by Hechmi Toumi

Contributors
Anand Kumar, Ana Oliveira, Ankit Sriwastava, Bhagyashree Parab, Devarshi Rastogi, Hechmi Toumi, Jia-Yun Chen, Jian-Feng Yang, Liliana Fonseca, Ram Lakhan Singh, Raquel Araújo, Ricardo Sousa, Sadaf Hasan, Samiya Khan, Sara Xavier Pires, Shah Waliullah, Shatakshi Pant, Sheila Jamal, Tomás Fonseca, Uday Raj, Virendra Pandey, Vivek Kumar Verma, Wen-Bin Zou, Xin-Ying Tang, Yuan-Chen Wang, Zeenat Ara, Zhuan Liao

First published in London, United Kingdom, 2026 by IntechOpen
IntechOpen is the global imprint of INTECHOPEN LIMITED, registered in England and Wales, registration number: 11086078, 167-169 Great Portland Street, London, W1W 5PF, United Kingdom

For EU product safety concerns: IN TECH d.o.o., Prolaz Marije Krucifikse Kozulić 3, 51000 Rijeka, Croatia, info@intechopen.com or visit our website at intechopen.com.

British Library Cataloguing-in-Publication Data
A catalogue record for this book is available from the British Library

Osteoporosis Overview - Importance of Screening and Treatment
Edited by Hechmi Toumi
p. cm.
Print ISBN 978-1-83635-514-4
Online ISBN 978-1-83635-513-7
eBook (PDF) ISBN 978-1-83635-515-1

Meet the editor

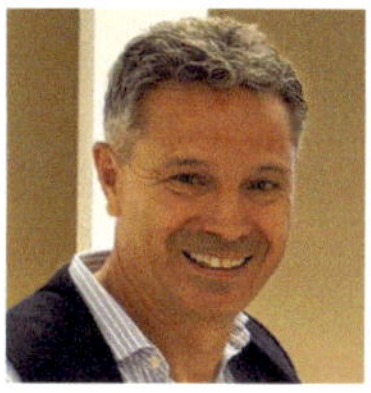

Professor Hechmi Toumi is a university professor, researcher, and international expert in gait analysis, musculoskeletal disorders, medical imaging, and physical exercise. He has held academic and research positions in France, the United States, and the United Kingdom, including at Cardiff University and the University of Orléans, where he served as Dean of the Faculty of Sciences from 2013 to 2018. His work focuses on movement analysis, anatomy, medical technology, and the prevention, diagnosis, and treatment of musculoskeletal conditions. Professor Toumi is an inventor with an international patent for algorithms that detect soft-tissue abnormalities on standard radiographs. He has authored scientific publications, served as editor and reviewer for international journals, and leads translational research initiatives at the University Hospital of Orléans, France.

Contents

Preface

Osteoporosis is one of the most common chronic skeletal diseases worldwide and represents a major public health challenge. Characterized by reduced bone strength and increased fracture risk, osteoporosis affects millions of individuals and is associated with substantial morbidity, mortality, loss of independence, and healthcare costs. Despite considerable advances in diagnosis and treatment, osteoporosis remains underdiagnosed and undertreated in many countries, highlighting the ongoing need for improved awareness, screening, prevention, and management strategies.

The aim of this book, *Osteoporosis Overview – Importance of Screening and Treatment*, is to provide readers with an up-to-date, comprehensive overview of current knowledge in osteoporosis. The chapters in this volume explore the epidemiology and burden of the disease, the biological mechanisms underlying bone fragility, current approaches to screening and fracture risk assessment, and established and emerging therapeutic strategies.

Particular attention is given to the importance of early diagnosis and timely intervention, which remain essential for reducing fracture risk and improving patient outcomes. The book also addresses specific clinical situations, secondary causes of osteoporosis, advances in imaging and diagnostic technologies, and future perspectives in personalized bone health management.

By bringing together contributions from experts across disciplines, this volume aims to provide clinicians, researchers, healthcare professionals, and students with practical, scientifically grounded information that can help improve the prevention and treatment of osteoporosis worldwide.

I would like to express my sincere gratitude to all contributing authors for sharing their expertise and valuable work. Their contributions have made this volume possible. I also thank the editorial team for their support throughout the preparation of this book.

I hope that readers will find this book informative, useful, and inspiring for both clinical practice and future research.

Hechmi Toumi
Professor,
Translational Medicine Research Platform (PRIMMO)
and Department of Rheumatology,
Orleans Hospital Center,
Faculty of Sciences and Technology,
University of Orleans,
Orleans, France

Chapter 1

Introductory Chapter: Confronting the Silent Epidemic of Osteoporosis Epidemiology and Clinical Burden

Hechmi Toumi

1. Introduction

Osteoporosis is one of the most prevalent chronic skeletal disorders worldwide and represents a major cause of fragility fractures, disability, and loss of independence among older adults. It is characterized by a progressive reduction in bone mineral density (BMD) and deterioration of bone microarchitecture, ultimately compromising bone strength and increasing susceptibility to fractures [1]. Often referred to as a "silent epidemic," osteoporosis typically remains asymptomatic until a fracture occurs, most commonly involving the wrist, hip, or spine [2].

It is estimated that nearly one in three women and one in five men worldwide will experience at least one osteoporotic fracture during their lifetime, with approximately 200 million individuals currently affected [3, 4]. Despite its major clinical consequences, osteoporosis remains substantially underdiagnosed and undertreated worldwide, even after the occurrence of fragility fractures. Indeed, many individuals are diagnosed only after the occurrence of a first fracture, reflecting important gaps in screening and preventive care.

The burden of osteoporosis extends far beyond bone fragility alone. Osteoporotic fractures are associated with chronic pain, impaired mobility, reduced quality of life, social isolation, institutionalization, and increased mortality. Hip fractures, in particular, are associated with a one-year mortality rate ranging from 8% to 36% [5]. Vertebral fractures, although sometimes clinically silent, can lead to progressive kyphosis, respiratory impairment, chronic pain, and substantial functional decline.

In addition to its clinical impact, osteoporosis represents a major socioeconomic challenge. The economic burden associated with hospitalization, surgery, rehabilitation, long-term care, and indirect societal costs is considerable and continues to increase worldwide [6]. With the progressive aging of the global population and increasing life expectancy, the incidence of osteoporotic fractures is expected to rise substantially over the coming decades. This demographic transition places considerable strain on healthcare systems worldwide and highlights the urgent need for effective prevention, early diagnosis, and long-term management strategies.

IntechOpen

2. Osteoporosis in men and secondary osteoporosis

Although osteoporosis is often perceived primarily as a disease affecting post-menopausal women, osteoporosis in men represents an increasingly recognized public health issue. Men account for a substantial proportion of osteoporotic fractures and often experience higher morbidity and mortality after hip fractures compared with women. However, osteoporosis in men remains underdiagnosed and under-treated, partly due to lower awareness and less frequent screening practices.

Secondary osteoporosis also contributes significantly to the global burden of skeletal fragility. Numerous medical conditions and treatments may adversely affect bone metabolism, including endocrine disorders, chronic inflammatory diseases, gastrointestinal malabsorption syndromes, chronic kidney disease, cancer therapies, and prolonged glucocorticoid use. Lifestyle-related factors such as smoking, alcohol consumption, physical inactivity, and poor nutrition further contribute to bone loss and fracture risk.

3. Pathophysiological mechanisms

At the biological level, bone health is maintained through a dynamic remodeling process involving the coordinated activity of osteoclast-mediated bone resorption and osteoblast-driven bone formation. This tightly regulated process ensures skeletal integrity and adaptation to mechanical stress throughout life. The receptor activator of nuclear factor kappa-B ligand (RANKL)–osteoprotegerin (OPG) signaling pathway plays a central role in regulating this balance [7]. Increased RANKL activity promotes osteoclast differentiation and activation, whereas OPG acts as a decoy receptor that inhibits osteoclastogenesis.

Disruption of this tightly regulated system results in increased bone resorption and reduced bone formation, ultimately leading to bone fragility. In postmenopausal women, estrogen deficiency is a major driver of this imbalance, leading to increased RANKL expression, enhanced osteoclast activity, and accelerated bone loss [8].

Beyond hormonal changes, osteoporosis is increasingly recognized as a multifactorial disease involving complex interactions between aging, inflammation, endocrine regulation, nutrition, genetics, and mechanical loading. Chronic low-grade inflammation associated with aging, often referred to as "inflammaging," contributes to increased osteoclast activity and impaired bone formation. Inflammatory cytokines such as TNF-α, IL-1, and IL-6 play important roles in bone resorption and skeletal deterioration.

Recent evidence has also highlighted the importance of osteocytes, which are now recognized as central regulators of bone remodeling and mechanosensing. Alterations in osteocyte function contribute to impaired skeletal adaptation and reduced bone quality with aging. Furthermore, bone strength depends not only on BMD but also on bone quality, including microarchitecture, collagen integrity, mineralization, and microdamage accumulation.

The relationship between bone and muscle health has also gained increasing attention in recent years. Sarcopenia and osteoporosis frequently coexist in older adults, giving rise to the concept of osteosarcopenia. Reduced muscle mass and function contribute to falls and fracture risk, while decreased mechanical loading negatively affects bone remodeling. This close interaction underscores the importance of integrated musculoskeletal approaches to healthy aging.

4. Importance of screening and early intervention

Given the asymptomatic nature of osteoporosis, early detection remains a major clinical challenge. Screening strategies based on BMD assessment and fracture risk evaluation are essential to identify individuals at high risk before fractures occur. Dual-energy X-ray absorptiometry (DXA) remains the gold standard for BMD assessment, while tools such as FRAX® facilitate estimation of fracture probability by integrating clinical risk factors.

Early identification of high-risk individuals enables timely intervention and may significantly reduce fracture incidence, morbidity, mortality, and healthcare costs. Preventive strategies include adequate calcium and vitamin D intake, regular weight-bearing exercise, fall prevention, smoking cessation, moderation of alcohol consumption, and maintenance of overall musculoskeletal health.

In recent years, increasing emphasis has been placed on personalized approaches to osteoporosis management. Advances in imaging techniques, biomarkers, artificial intelligence, and fracture risk prediction models are progressively improving diagnostic precision and therapeutic decision-making. In parallel, novel pharmacological therapies targeting bone resorption and bone formation continue to expand therapeutic possibilities.

Despite these advances, major challenges remain regarding patient adherence, long-term treatment persistence, and implementation of effective fracture liaison services. Improving awareness among healthcare professionals and the general population, therefore, remains essential to reducing the burden of osteoporotic fractures worldwide.

5. Conclusion

Osteoporosis represents a complex and multifactorial disease that requires a comprehensive and multidisciplinary approach. Understanding its epidemiology, biological mechanisms, clinical implications, and evolving therapeutic strategies is essential for improving patient outcomes and addressing the growing global burden of this condition.

By integrating epidemiological, biological, clinical, and preventive perspectives, this introductory chapter provides the conceptual framework necessary for understanding current advances and future challenges in osteoporosis research, diagnosis, prevention, and patient care. The following sections of this volume will further explore these dimensions, with particular emphasis on emerging mechanisms, innovative diagnostic approaches, and evolving therapeutic strategies aimed at improving skeletal health and reducing fracture risk across the lifespan.

Acknowledgment of AI-assisted language editing

The author acknowledges the use of ChatGPT (OpenAI, San Francisco, CA, USA) for language polishing, grammar correction, and improvement of the academic writing style of the manuscript. The author takes full responsibility for the scientific content, interpretation, and conclusions presented in this work.

Author details

Hechmi Toumi[1,2,3,4]

1 Translational Medicine Research Platform, PRIMMO, University Hospital Center of Orleans, Orleans, France

2 Department of Rheumatology, University Hospital Center of Orleans, Orleans, France

3 University of Orleans, Orleans, France

4 Laboratory des Adaptations Métaboliques à l'Exercice en conditions Physiologiques et Pathologiques (AME2P), UCA University, Clermont Ferrand, Aubière, France

*Address all correspondence to: hechmi.toumi@chu-orleans.fr

References

[1] National Institutes of Health Consensus Development Panel. Osteoporosis prevention, diagnosis, and therapy. Journal of the American Medical Association. 2001;**285**(6):785-795

[2] Kanis JA, Cooper C, Rizzoli R, Reginster JY. Scientific Advisory Board of the European Society for Clinical and Economic Aspects of Osteoporosis (ESCEO) and the committees of scientific advisors and National Societies of the international osteoporosis foundation (IOF). European guidance for the diagnosis and management of osteoporosis in postmenopausal women. Osteoporosis International. 2019;**30**(1):3-44

[3] International Osteoporosis Foundation. Epidemiology of osteoporosis and fragility fractures. Archives of Osteoporosis. 2021;**16**(1):82

[4] Salari N, Ghasemi H, Mohammadi L, Rabieenia E, Shohaimi S, Mohammadi M, et al. The global prevalence of osteoporosis in the world: A comprehensive systematic review and meta-analysis. Journal of Orthopaedic Surgery and Research. 2021;**16**(1):609

[5] Haentjens P, Magaziner J, Colón-Emeric CS, Vanderschueren D, Milisen K, Velkeniers B, et al. Meta-analysis: Excess mortality after hip fracture among older women and men. Annals of Internal Medicine. 2010;**152**(6):380-390

[6] Burge R, Dawson-Hughes B, Solomon DH, Wong JB, King A, Tosteson A. Incidence and economic burden of osteoporosis-related fractures in the United States, 2005-2025. Journal of Bone and Mineral Research. 2007;**22**(3):465-475

[7] Boyce BF, Xing L. Functions of RANKL/RANK/OPG in bone modeling and remodeling. Archives of Biochemistry and Biophysics. 2008;**473**(2):139-146

[8] Khosla S, Oursler MJ, Monroe DG. Estrogen and the skeleton. Trends in Endocrinology and Metabolism. 2012;**23**(11):576-581

Chapter 2

Osteoporosis: Its Pathophysiology, Diagnosis and Role of Nutraceuticals in Its Management

Shah Waliullah, Zeenat Ara, Ankit Sriwastava, Vivek Kumar Verma, Anand Kumar, Devarshi Rastogi, Shatakshi Pant, Virendra Pandey, Uday Raj and Ram Lakhan Singh

Abstract

Osteoporosis is a classical age-related metabolic bone disorder that affects women more commonly than men. The disease is primarily characterized by low bone mass and alterations in the microstructure of bone, which often result in increased fragility. Iron also plays a significant role in the human body; however, its abnormal metabolism, known as iron overload, is another significant factor contributing to the pathophysiology of Osteoporosis. In recent years, nutraceuticals such as phytoestrogens, micronutrients, macronutrients, and vitamins have garnered considerable attention due to their ease of consumption, cost-effectiveness, and beneficial properties, including antioxidant, anti-inflammatory, and anti-ageing effects. These properties help slow the progression of Osteoporosis, enhance bone mineralization and thereby reduce the risk of fracture. Although Osteoporosis cannot be cured, adopting a healthy lifestyle, a balanced diet and using nutritional supplements are important factors in its prevention.

Keywords: osteoporosis, BMD, ROS, fracture, oestrogen, RANKL, osteoprotegerin, phytoestrogen, nutraceuticals, mineralization, standard deviation, fracture, postmenopausal, hip, wrist, spine, denosumab injection, senile, primary, RANKL, oxidative stress

1. Introduction

Osteoporosis is a common skeletal disorder characterized by a gradual decrease in bone mineral density, resulting in compromised bone strength and increased fragility, making bones more susceptible to fractures. These fractures often occur after minimal trauma and most frequently involve the wrist, hip, and spine. With the steady rise in the ageing population, osteoporosis has emerged as an important public health problem worldwide. Bone strength depends not only on bone mineral density but also on bone quality, including factors such as bone microarchitecture and turnover.

Studies have shown that even a one standard deviation (SD) reduction in BMD is associated with a marked increase in fracture risk. According to the International Osteoporosis Foundation (IOF, 2021), osteoporosis is currently ranked as the fourth most burdensome chronic disease globally, after ischemic heart disease, dementia, and lung cancer. Although Osteoporosis is most prevalent among postmenopausal women, it is not limited to this group and can affect men and individuals of all ages. The IOF estimates that nearly one-third of women and one-fifth of men will suffer at least one fragility fracture during their lifetime [1, 2].

Several risk factors contribute to the development of Osteoporosis, including ageing, poor dietary habits, menopause, long-term glucocorticoid therapy, and inherited conditions such as osteogenesis imperfecta. The disorder is broadly classified into primary and secondary Osteoporosis. Primary Osteoporosis, which is most common in postmenopausal women, is further divided into Type 1 (postmenopausal), primarily caused by oestrogen deficiency, and Type 2 (senile), which arises from age-related systemic changes.

Currently, Osteoporosis is treated with several pharmacological options, including bisphosphonates, denosumab, teriparatide, and vitamin D supplementation. These therapies primarily work by modulating the biological pathways that regulate bone remodelling and bone turnover. In recent years, increasing attention has been given to their effects on immune-related mediators involved in bone metabolism. In postmenopausal women, reduced oestrogen levels play a key role in disturbing normal bone homeostasis. Oestrogen deficiency leads to an altered balance between receptor activator of nuclear factor-κB ligand (RANKL) and osteoprotegerin (OPG), with higher RANKL expression and a relative reduction in OPG. As a result, osteoclast activity increases, favouring bone resorption over bone formation and ultimately causing bone loss. Similar alterations in the RANKL–OPG system have been described in several disease conditions. These include rheumatoid arthritis, multiple myeloma and osteolytic metastatic bone disease. A comparable mechanism is also seen in patients with prostate cancer receiving androgen deprivation therapy and in breast cancer patients treated with aromatase inhibitors, where treatment-induced hormonal changes negatively affect bone health [1–4].

Denosumab, a fully human monoclonal antibody, specifically targets RANKL, thereby preventing the maturation and differentiation of pre-osteoclasts and promoting osteoclast apoptosis. In this way, it exerts a potent anti-resorptive effect. The pivotal FREEDOM Phase III clinical trial demonstrated that denosumab effectively reduces the risk of vertebral, nonvertebral, and hip fractures in postmenopausal women with Osteoporosis. Notably, improvements in femoral neck BMD were significantly correlated with reduced fracture risk [5–7].

Long-term data reveal that denosumab maintains continuous efficacy for at least 10 years, preventing both vertebral and nonvertebral fractures, and improving lumbar spine and proximal femoral BMD. Importantly, unlike oral bisphosphonates, denosumab also produces a linear increase in BMD at the 1/3 radius, a site predominantly composed of cortical bone [7, 8].

The FREEDOM extension study further showed that prolonged treatment with denosumab reduces the annual incidence of nonvertebral fractures. During the first 3 years of therapy, the incidence exceeded 2%, but declined to below 2% after 4 to 7 years, and reached 0.7% after 8 years of continuous use [9].

Pharmacokinetically, denosumab is primarily cleared by the reticuloendothelial system, with minimal renal excretion and no hepatic metabolism. As circulating concentrations decline, bone resorption markers rise within 4 months, continuing to increase until the next scheduled injection at 6 months. Following discontinuation, increased RANKL expression at sites of microdamage may trigger bone remodelling; however, this remains an area for further investigation [8].

As denosumab inhibits RANKL-induced resorption, patients must receive adequate vitamin D and calcium supplementation to reduce the risk of hypocalcaemia, particularly within the first week of administration. Long-term therapy has also been associated with rare but serious adverse effects, including atypical femoral fractures and osteonecrosis of the jaw. Upon discontinuation, a rapid rebound increase in bone turnover may occur, leading to substantial bone loss and an increased risk of fractures. Therefore, it is recommended that discontinuation of denosumab be followed by an alternative anti-resorptive therapy [10–12].

2. Epidemiology of Osteoporosis

Vertebral fractures are considered the most common type of osteoporotic fracture worldwide, particularly in individuals over 50 years of age. Several studies indicate that between 30 and 50% of people in this age group are affected, although many cases remain undiagnosed. Women who have already experienced a vertebral fracture are at a markedly increased risk of future fractures. The likelihood of sustaining another vertebral fracture is almost four times higher, while the risk of non-vertebral fractures increases by approximately 1.5 to 2 times. Importantly, this risk continues to rise with both the number and severity of existing fractures. Advancing age further contributes to this burden. Around 25% of women aged 75 years have at least one vertebral fracture, and by 80 years of age, this figure approaches 50%. Overall, the estimated lifetime prevalence of vertebral fractures ranges from 30 to 50% in women and 20–30% in men. Indian studies reflect a similar pattern. The reported overall prevalence of vertebral fractures in India is 17.9%, with rates of 18.8% in men and 17.1% in women, values that are comparable to those observed in Western populations [2, 3]. In contrast, higher prevalence rates have been reported in specific subgroups. For example, Nongkynrih B documented a prevalence of 30.4% among rural postmenopausal women, highlighting the considerable burden in this population [3, 4].

Hip fractures account for 329,000 of 1.5 million annual osteoporotic fractures in the USA, with 10–24% mortality within a year [5]. Rates are the highest in the USA and Northern Europe, the lowest in Africa and Latin America, and intermediate in Asia. By 2050, cases are projected to exceed 6 million [6, 7].

Distal radius fractures (DRFs), the most common upper extremity fractures in the elderly—especially women—have increased 17% in the USA over 40 years, and nearly doubled in Sweden's older population over 30 years [7, 8]. In Korea, surgical management of DRFs rose from 32.6% in 2011 to 38.3% in 2015, reflecting the growing global burden of osteoporotic fractures and their health care costs [2–6].

3. Economic burden

Fractures place a heavy burden on healthcare. By 2025, Osteoporosis is expected to cause nearly 3 million fractures in the USA, costing $25.3 billion annually. Hip fractures, about 14% of all fractures, account for up to 72% of treatment costs. In the year after a fracture, average US healthcare expenses are $17,000, while Canada spends $1.1 billion annually on hip fractures in adults over 65.

In the USA, Osteoporosis causes over 1.5 million vertebral fractures each year, resulting in 500,000 hospitalizations, 800,000 emergency visits, and 2.6 million physician visits, with costs of $12–18 billion. However, data on the direct economic burden of osteoporotic fractures in India remain scarce.

3.1 Consideration of targets in Osteoporosis

The World Health Organisation (WHO) defines Osteoporosis as a condition characterized by a T-score of ≤ -2.5 standard deviations (SD) as measured by dual-energy X-ray absorptiometry (DXA). Hip fractures are associated with a substantially increased one-year mortality rate, ranging from 8 to 36%, with the higher rates observed in men. Furthermore, hip fractures confer a 2.5-fold elevated risk of subsequent fractures. Approximately 20% of affected patients require long-term nursing care, and only 40% regain their pre-fracture level of independence [13, 14]. While most vertebral fractures are initially asymptomatic, they frequently result in pain, disability, deformity, and increased mortality over time [13–16]. In the 1980s, Riggs and Melton identified two separate types of involutional Osteoporosis: postmenopausal Osteoporosis (type 1) and senile Osteoporosis (type 2).

Type 1 Osteoporosis, associated with menopause, is characterized by rapid trabecular bone loss occurring predominantly in the decade following oestrogen deficiency [17]. Conversely, type 2 osteoporosis, which is more prevalent among older men, involves a gradual loss of both trabecular and cortical bone, primarily attributable to osteoblast dysfunction. In 1998, this dualistic model was superseded by the "unitary model" of Osteoporosis, which encompasses both postmenopausal women and ageing men [18].

In this model, oestrogen deficiency is the primary driver of bone loss in postmenopausal women and also contributes to Osteoporosis in older men. Hyperthyroidism, from whether primary thyroid disease or long-term/over-replacement levothyroxine therapy, accelerates bone turnover, lowers bone mineral density (BMD) and increases hip and vertebral fracture risk. By contrast, hypothyroidism slows bone turnover without raising fracture risk, though subclinical hypothyroidism in postmenopausal women is linked to lower BMD and higher fracture risk [19].

The UK National Institute for Health and Care Excellence (NICE) advises that risk assessment be conducted for all women aged 65 and above, men aged 75 and above, and younger patients with risk factors. BMD remains the gold standard, and the FRAX score utilizes femoral neck BMD, age, sex, smoking status, family history (e.g., parental hip fracture), and glucocorticoid use to estimate the 10-year probability of fracture. In 2020, the International Osteoporosis Foundation (IOF) and ESCEO introduced an algorithm to further stratify patients into high- and very high-risk groups [20–22].

The availability of anabolic agents—new options such as abaloparatide and romosozumab, along with teriparatide—has advanced osteoporosis therapy. Teriparatide is more effective than antiresorptive drugs in reducing fracture risk [23–26].

NICE, NOGG and IOF/ESCEO guidelines suggest that oral bisphosphonates should be the first-line treatment for women at high risk. In contrast, patients classified as very high risk might gain more from initiating treatment with anabolic therapy, which should then be followed by resorption inhibitors. Typically, anabolic agents are prescribed for an duration of 12 to 24 months, after which their effectiveness tends to diminish. Nevertheless, when these agents are used in conjunction with turnover inhibitors, their positive effects on bone mineral density (BMD) and fracture risk can continue. Research indicates that this treatment sequence is more effective in preventing fractures compared to the reverse order [25–28].

Taiwan's ageing population has led to a sharp rise in Osteoporosis, reflecting broader Asian trends. Both Asian and Caucasian groups are considered high risk, although Taiwan's epidemiology may differ due to its unique demographics [29].

Fracture incidence varies geographically and is influenced by skeletal size. With increasing age, osteoporosis and fractures—most commonly hip fractures—become more frequent. Data from Taiwan's National Health Insurance (NHI) and the Ministry of Health indicate that the number of hip fractures rose from 15,668 in 2001 to 21,775 in 2012. The incidence rates were consistent from 2001 to 2005, ranging between 333 and 337 per 100,000 person-years, but fell to 296 per 100,000 by 2012 [28].

NHI inpatient data show that hip fractures in men over 50 rose from 3551 in 1999 to 8616 in 2010, and in women from 6096 to 13,893, representing an annual increase of 9.3%. Although the prevalence of Osteoporosis declined slightly in those over 70, the population aged 50 and above increased from 4.3 to 6.9 million, resulting in more fractures [30].

Among fracture types, intertrochanteric fractures (51.6%) slightly exceed femoral neck fractures (48.4%). Risks are higher in individuals with chronic diseases such as diabetes, rheumatoid arthritis, stroke, Parkinson's disease, cancer, and organ transplant, and those undergoing dialysis. A meta-analysis revealed that a decrease in hip BMD of one standard deviation increased the risk of hip fractures by 2.6-fold and other fractures by 1.6-fold [28, 30].

Ethnicity also influences bone mass: African Americans, who have higher BMD, experience lower osteoporosis rates than Caucasians. Chinese BMD is similar to or slightly lower than that of Caucasians. The Global Burden of Disease study reports lower T-scores in Asia, with Asian ethnicity associated with lower BMD even after adjusting for BMI.

The T-score is determined by subtracting the bone mineral density (BMD) of the reference population—typically a healthy 30-year-old individual, representing peak bone mass and maximal fracture risk—from the subject's BMD. This difference is then divided by the standard deviation (SD) of the reference population's BMD values. Mathematically, the T-score is expressed as: T-score (BMD-YN)/SD.

3.2 Risk factors for Osteoporosis

Non-modifiable risk factors consist of genetic predisposition, increased longevity and ethnicity. In contrast, modifiable risk factors include deficiencies in calcium and vitamin D, often resulting from low calcium intake, sociocultural influences that restrict sunlight exposure, insufficient vitamin D fortification in food products and the presence of highly pigmented skin. Moreover, other modifiable factors include a high intake of phytates and oxalates, which are common in the Indian diet, and can impede calcium absorption. Other contributing factors include early menopause, a sedentary lifestyle, low levels of physical activity, a lack of awareness regarding bone health and a history of fractures.

3.3 Risk factor of Osteoporosis in India

In 2015, it was anticipated that 230 million Indians would be around 50 years of age, with 20% expected to sustain osteoporotic fractures. Women of all ethnic groups are more susceptible to low bone mass after menopause, primarily due to the vital role of the oestrogen hormone in bone formation and growth. Additionally, Indian women experience menopause approximately 10 years earlier than Caucasian women.

Genetic factors are significantly associated with bone mass, and Indian women generally exhibit lower bone mineral density (BMD) compared to other ethnic groups. Some researchers speculate that vitamin D receptor polymorphisms may be responsible for the varying results observed.

Vitamin D is crucial for gut health as it promotes calcium absorption and helps maintain adequate serum calcium levels, both of which are essential for normal bone mineralization. Furthermore, vitamin D plays a crucial role in bone growth and remodelling by regulating the activity of osteoblasts and osteoclasts. Vitamin D deficiency is defined as having 25(OH)D levels below 50 nmol/L and can lead to increased bone turnover, bone loss and a higher risk of osteoporotic fractures. A meta-analysis by Tang et al. indicated that a daily intake of at least 800 IU of vitamin D enhances calcium absorption and is associated with a 3% reduction in total fracture risk compared to lower daily intakes.

In a 6-year cohort study involving 773 senior Japanese women, Nakamura et al. demonstrated that sufficient vitamin D levels (greater than 71 nmol/L) were associated with a 58% reduction in the occurrence of osteoporotic fractures compared to subjects with vitamin D deficiency. This study concluded that maintaining adequate vitamin D levels can help reduce the risk of osteoporotic fractures.

Vitamin D receptors (VDRs), located on osteoblasts, osteoclasts and osteocytes, regulate bone remodelling to maintain skeletal health. A meta-analysis has shown that vitamin D supplementation can decrease the incidence of falls.

The quality of the skeleton is determined by bone remodelling, a process that maintains a balance between bone resorption (carried out by osteoclasts) and bone formation (conducted by osteoblasts). Various molecules influence this balance. Osteoblasts originate from mesenchymal stem cells and progenitor cells, and their activity and survival are promoted by various factors, including bone morphogenetic proteins, transforming growth factor-β, Wnt proteins, insulin, neurotransmitters, fibroblast growth factors, and parathyroid hormone.

These factors bind to intracellular signalling molecules, activating various transcription factors. A critical factor for osteoblast differentiation is the Runt-related transcription factor 2. This process leads to the release of type I collagen (COL I) and other proteins that comprise the bone matrix. Osteoblasts also produce both positive and negative regulators of osteoclastogenesis, such as the nuclear factor (NF)-κB ligand (RANKL) and the natural decoy receptor for RANKL, and osteoprotegerin (OPG), respectively. Conversely, negative regulators such as Dickkopf-related protein one and sclerostin, primarily produced by osteocytes, disrupt the Wnt signalling pathway, thereby inhibiting osteoblast function. Additionally, cytokines such as interleukin-6 (IL-6) and tumour necrosis factor-alpha (TNF-α) also inhibit osteoblast activity.

The RANKL decoy receptor OPG is one of the negative regulators of osteoclastogenesis. It is produced not only by osteoblast cells but also by B lymphocytes and dendritic cells. Other negative regulators include interferon-γ, IL-3, IL-4, IL-10 and IL-12.In 2015, it was anticipated that 230 million Indians would be around 50 years of age, with 20% expected to sustain osteoporotic fractures. Women of all ethnic groups are more susceptible to low bone mass after menopause, primarily due to the vital role of the oestrogen hormone in bone formation and growth. Additionally, Indian women experience menopause approximately 10 years earlier than Caucasian women.

4. History and physical examination

A comprehensive patient history, which includes medical conditions, long-term medication use, dietary habits and familial occurrences of fragility fractures—particularly on the maternal side—can provide valuable insights into the underlying causes of Osteoporosis. Fractures can lead to chronic pain, decreased mobility, disability, dependence and even mortality. Observable signs such as loss of height (commonly resulting from vertebral compression), dorsal kyphosis, chest deformities, a protruding abdomen and rib-pelvic overlap may suggest the presence of vertebral fractures. These physical changes can compress internal organs, resulting in symptoms such as diminished appetite, early satiety, constipation and abdominal pain. Persistent back pain and difficulty finding comfortable positions are commonplace. Additionally, factors such as impaired ambulation, muscle weakness, poor balance, vision impairment and orthostatic hypotension significantly increase the risk of falls and subsequent fractures.

4.1 Laboratory investigation

Recommended laboratory investigations include a complete blood count (CBC), serum creatinine with estimated glomerular filtration rate (eGFR), and serum levels of calcium, phosphorus, magnesium, alkaline phosphatase, alanine aminotransferase (ALT), aspartate aminotransferase (AST), thyroid-stimulating hormone (TSH), serum protein electrophoresis, 25-hydroxy vitamin D (25-OH-D), total testosterone and gonadotropins in younger male patients, in addition to biochemical turnover markers (BTMs). Vitamin D status should be reassessed 3 to 4 months after supplementation; if serum 25-OH-D concentrations reach ≥30 ng/mL, further testing may not be necessary. More extensive diagnostic evaluations are recommended for men who present with unexplained fractures, low bone mineral density (BMD), inadequate therapeutic response or suspected secondary Osteoporosis. These assessments may encompass the measurements of iron and ferritin levels, homocysteine, prolactin, tryptase, urinary histamine and urine protein electrophoresis.

4.2 Non-pharmacological treatment

Vitamin D deficiency in India is prevalent due to several factors, including limited sun exposure, traditional clothing, darker skin tones, poor dietary habits and a lack of fortified foods. These factors hinder calcium absorption and bone mineralization. Individuals who have been using corticosteroids for an extended period should receive calcium and vitamin D supplementation. Adopting lifestyle changes, such as regular exercise, quitting smoking, and moderate alcohol consumption, can enhance bone health and lower the risk of fractures.

Effective lifestyle management is essential and includes maintaining a balanced diet, engaging in regular physical activity, and ensuring adequate exposure to sunlight. It is advisable to avoid tobacco and alcohol. Sodium intake should be limited to less than 5 grams per day, protein consumption should be around 1 gram per kilogramme of body weight, and caffeine intake should be restricted to fewer than 3 cups daily. It is recommended that calcium intake exceeds 800 mg per day; however, supplements may be necessary for additional support. Certain medications, such as thyroid drugs, corticosteroids, tetracyclines, anticonvulsants, and iron supplements, may interfere with calcium absorption. For treating deficiency, a dose of cholecalciferol 60,000 IU weekly for 8 weeks (taken with milk) or a single intramuscular dose of 600,000 IU is suggested; the latter should not be repeated within 3 months. For maintenance, a dose of 60,000 IU monthly during summer or twice monthly during winter can be considered, or intramuscular injections of 300,000 IU twice a year or 600,000 IU once a year may be administered.

5. Indian menopausal society guidelines

For early postmenopausal women without contraindications, oestrogen-progesterone therapy (EPT) or oestrogen therapy (ET) is recommended for the prevention and management of symptoms (Grade A). Progestogens should be included in ET for women with a uterus to reduce the risk of endometrial hyperplasia (Grade B). A comprehensive evaluation for menopausal hormone therapy (MHT) is essential, along with annual follow-ups, gynaecological assessments, breast self-examinations, clinical breast examinations yearly and mammograms every 1 to 3 years (Grade C) [29, 30].

Calcitonin, a peptide hormone that inhibits osteoclasts, helps reduce bone loss. Salmon calcitonin (200 IU intranasally once daily) is the most commonly used form. It is typically administered in conjunction with calcium and vitamin D, particularly for managing vertebral crush fractures or when other treatments are not suitable. The benefits include pain relief in vertebral fractures, though side effects may include rhinitis, nosebleeds and allergic reactions. Despite these, it remains useful in selected cases [29–31].

Osteoclasts, which originate from monocyte/macrophage precursors, share pathways with immune cells. Interactions between the immune system and bone cells drive bone destruction in conditions such as periodontitis and rheumatoid arthritis (RA). CD4+ T cells, particularly Th17 cells, play a critical role in RA, as they promote osteoclastogenesis by inducing RANKL expression in synovial fibroblasts through the action of IL-17. IL-17 further increases levels of TNF and IL-6, stimulating osteoclast activity. Oestrogen deficiency increases osteoclast numbers while decreasing osteoblast activity, leading to a shift in bone remodelling towards resorption. This occurs indirectly through pro-osteoclastogenic cytokines (TNF, IL-1, IL-6 and IL-17), which show a significant rise in the first 10 years after menopause, highlighting their role in the development of Osteoporosis [30–32].

5.1 The impact of inflammation on bone cells

During inflammation, immune cells—including T cells, B cells, macrophages and dendritic cells—are activated, and they release cytokines, which play a critical role in osteoimmunology.

T cells play a vital role in promoting osteoclastogenesis through cytokines such as TNF-α and RANKL, thereby contributing significantly to the progression of Osteoporosis. By the 1980s, TNF-α and IL-1 were recognized as the potent stimulators of bone resorption and inhibitors of bone formation. IL-6, another significant pro-resorptive cytokine, is commonly found in circulation and exhibits high activity. In combination with RANKL, TNF-α, IL-6, and IL-1 enhance osteoclast activity while inhibiting osteoblast function.

Additionally, TNF-α facilitates bone resorption indirectly by stimulating M-CSF in bone marrow stromal cells and decreasing osteoblast-derived OPG. IL-17 further contributes to bone loss by increasing levels of RANKL. Research has shown that oestrogen deficiency leads to increased IL-1 production in mononuclear cells, while additional studies have indicated RANKL upregulation in early postmenopausal women.

Furthermore, osteoporotic women with fractures tend to have a higher expression of TNF-α in CD8+ cells compared to the control group. Ageing is also associated with chronic, low-grade inflammation, referred to as inflamm-ageing. This state is driven by excess cytokine production from macrophages and contributes to Osteoporosis, as well as age-related diseases, including atherosclerosis, dementia and sarcopenia.

5.2 Iron overload

Iron overload is clinically established when transferrin saturation (TSAT) levels exceed 40%, resulting from excessive iron accumulation in tissues. This condition can be classified as primary, stemming from genetic mutations that disrupt iron metabolism (such as HJV and TFR2), or secondary, often associated with haematological disorders like hereditary haemochromatosis (HH), thalassaemia and sickle cell anaemia (SCA). Additionally, long-term blood transfusions can contribute to secondary iron overload. Research by Nicolas et al. demonstrated that the overexpression of HAMP can reduce iron deposition in mouse models of HH and β-thalassaemia, underscoring the critical role of hepcidin regulation in both forms of the condition. Evidence from clinical trials suggests that excessive iron intake may contribute to the progression of Osteoporosis. Animal studies corroborate these findings, with mice suffering from thalassaemia and SCA exhibiting compromised bone characteristics consistent with clinical observations.

Stimulatory	Osteoblasts	Osteoclast
	BMPs (bone morphogenetic protein)	IL-1
	FGFs (fibroblast growth factor)	IL-6
	Insulin	IL-17
	PTH	M-CSF
	TGF beta	RANKL
	Wnt	TNF-α)
Inhibitory	**Osteoblast**	**Osteoclast**
	DKK1 (Dikkopf-related protein)	IFN gamma
	Interlukin 6	IL-3
	Interlukin 1	IL-4
	SOST(Sclerostin)	IL-10
	Tumour necrosis factor alpha	IL-12
		OIP 1
		OPG

Source: Pietschmann et al. [33].

Table 1.
Selected regulators of bone remodelling.

Liu et al. established a mouse model of iron overload using intraperitoneal injections of ferric ammonium citrate (FAC), revealing that this overload leads to classic symptoms of Osteoporosis, such as significant trabecular bone resorption and fractures. In summary, both clinical trials and animal studies have confirmed that excessive iron can disrupt the delicate equilibrium of bone remodelling, contributing to the onset of Osteoporosis.

The development of Osteoporosis is closely connected to mesenchymal stem cells, osteoblasts and osteoclasts. The primary mechanisms through which iron overload influences this condition include oxidative stress and ferritin autophagy, among others. Numerous pathways are implicated in this process. Iron overload disrupts bone remodelling by impairing the function of mesenchymal stem cells, osteoblasts and osteoclasts, with mechanisms such as oxidative stress, ferritin autophagy and related signalling pathways collectively disturbing the balance between bone formation and resorption, thereby promoting the progression of Osteoporosis (**Table 1**).

6. The diagnosis of osteoporosis involves two primary methods: Biohumoral and instrumental diagnostics

Biohumoral diagnosis focuses on specific biomarkers linked to bone health. For instance, in diabetic patients, serum osteocalcin levels negatively correlate with glucose concentrations and advanced glycation end products, which hurt bone metabolism. Thyroid disorders, particularly thyrotoxicosis, also significantly influence bone turnover, as receptors for thyroid-stimulating hormone (TSH) are found in both osteoblasts and osteoclasts [30–32].

In patients who have undergone thyroidectomy and are on L-thyroxine therapy, low TSH levels lead to increased osteoprotegerin (OPG) and decreased receptor activator of nuclear factor κB ligand (RANKL), contributing to an imbalance that is closely associated with vertebral fractures [32].

The liver and kidneys play crucial roles in clearing bone markers, and their dysfunction can alter the levels of these biomarkers. A decrease in glomerular filtration rate, for instance, leads to diminished urinary excretion of carboxy-terminal cross-linked telopeptides of type I collagen (CTX), resulting in elevated serum CTX concentrations [34].

Furthermore, biomarker levels can be affected by states of prolonged immobility, such as bed rest or microgravity, which lead to significant bone loss due to increased bone resorption and suppressed bone formation. Following a fracture, there is a marked increase in bone turnover markers within the first few weeks, which can persist for up to a year, depending on the severity of the fracture and the patient's age. Specifically, after minor fractures, such as forearm fractures, these markers may remain elevated for approximately 6 months, while markers after hip fractures can remain elevated for up to a year. Over time, however, bone turnover marker levels gradually decrease, underscoring the importance of monitoring them in the diagnosis and management of osteoporosis [34].

6.1 Role of nutrition in osteoporosis

Nutrition is widely recognized as an important factor in both the prevention and management of osteoporosis. Among the various nutrients, calcium and vitamin D have received the most attention due to their direct role in maintaining bone health. Several studies have shown that individuals with a higher lifetime calcium intake tend to have better bone mineral density (BMD). In postmenopausal women, in particular, adequate intake of calcium, along with vitamin D, is associated with slower bone loss, reduced bone turnover and a lower risk of non-vertebral fractures (**Figure 1**) [35].

Apart from calcium and vitamin D, potassium also plays a meaningful role in maintaining bone health. One of its primary functions is to help regulate calcium balance in the body, particularly by influencing the amount of calcium lost through the kidneys. When dietary potassium intake is low, urinary calcium loss tends to increase, which can have an adverse effect on bone health over time. Potassium is mainly obtained from foods such as fruits, vegetables, legumes and dairy products. Many of these foods also have an alkalising effect, which helps counteract dietary acid load. Previous research has reported links between net endogenous acid production (NEAP), potassium intake and bone mineral density, suggesting that sufficient potassium intake may contribute to better skeletal health [30–32, 34, 36, 37].

Additionally, a high-sodium diet has been shown to increase urinary calcium loss. Research suggests that in postmenopausal women, such a diet can lead to an increased rate of bone resorption over a four-week period. However, potassium-rich foods, including potassium citrate, have been found to mitigate these adverse effects. Furthermore, the consumption of fruits and vegetables high in potassium has been associated with greater baseline BMD and reduced bone loss [30–32, 34, 36, 37].

A recent study investigated the association between serum vitamin K1 levels and bone mineral density (BMD) in postmenopausal women diagnosed with Osteoporosis. The cohort comprised 23 postmenopausal osteoporotic subjects and 15 age-matched healthy controls. Serum vitamin K1 concentrations were quantified *via* enzyme-linked immunosorbent assay (ELISA), while lumbar spine BMD was

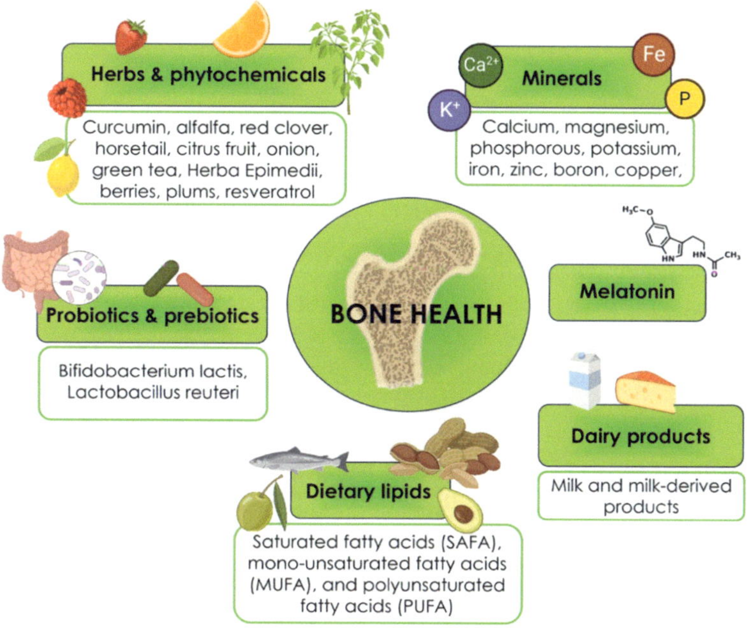

Figure 1.
Nutrients essential for bone health.

Nutrient	Recommended dietary allowance	Median intake
Vitamin D	600–800 IU	150–300 IU
Calcium	1000–1200 mg	735 mg
Magnesium	320–420 mg	243 mg
Silicon	*40 mg for bone health	21 mg
Vitamin K	90–120 ugm	70–80 umg
Boron	*3 mg for bone Health	1 mg
Vitamin C	75–90 mg	103 mg
Copper	0.9 mg	1.1 mg
Zinc	8-11 mg	9.6 mg
Manganese	1.8–2.3 mg	2.8 mg

Suggested intake (not standardized).

Table 2.
Recommended dietary allowance of various nutrients.

evaluated using standard densitometric techniques. The findings revealed that mean serum vitamin K1 levels were markedly reduced in the osteoporotic group compared to controls (0.794 vs. 3.61 ng/mL, $p < 0.0001$). Additionally, a significant positive correlation was observed between serum vitamin K1 concentrations and lumbar spine BMD in both osteoporotic patients ($R = 0.533$, $p = 0.009$) and healthy participants ($R = 0.563$, $p = 0.02$). These results underscore the potential role of vitamin K1 in modulating bone mineral density and highlight its prospective utility as a therapeutic target or diagnostic biomarker in the management of postmenopausal Osteoporosis (**Table 2**).

7. Common nutrients for bone health

7.1 Taurine and osteoporosis

Taurine and Osteoporosis: Individuals with Osteoporosis exhibit lower serum taurine levels compared to healthy subjects. Additionally, decreased urinary taurine serves as an indicator of both postmenopausal status and Osteoporosis; specifically, urinary taurine concentrations are approximately 1.9 times lower in postmenopausal women with Osteoporosis than in premenopausal women with normal bone mineral density (BMD) [1].

Treatment with bisphosphonates has been shown to elevate taurine levels in those with Osteoporosis. Research involving ovariectomized mice demonstrated that the administration of alendronate sodium, a type of bisphosphonate, raised taurine levels from 467.6 ± 116.0 μM to 669.2 ± 127.6 μM. Moreover, the uptake of taurine by retinal capillary endothelial cells, assessed through [^{3}H] labelling, was significantly enhanced following pretreatment with alendronate and pamidronate. *In vitro* experiments further revealed that alendronate, which mimics taurine's activity, can inhibit osteoclast formation stimulated by bacterial factors [1].

In another study, rabbits fed an atherogenic diet and supplemented with taurine exhibited normalized hyperhomocysteinaemia [1]. Similarly, taurine supplementation in humans has been shown to increase the activities of cystathionine β-synthase and cystathionine γ-lyase, two enzymes involved in the transsulfuration pathway. This enzymatic upregulation contributed to the reduction of plasma homocysteine (Hcy) levels, thereby suggesting an indirect role for taurine in preventing Osteoporosis.

Taurine, a polyfunctional molecule, plays a pivotal role in maintaining intracellular calcium homeostasis. Although serum calcium concentrations may remain within normal limits, taurine deficiency disrupts calcium handling in both osteoblasts and osteoclasts. This disruption impairs osteoblast activity, leading to reduced bone formation, while concurrently augmenting osteoclast-mediated bone resorption. Taurine is present in high concentrations in bone tissue, where it supports osteoblast function and helps mitigate excessive resorption. Taken together, these observations support taurine as a key regulator of bone growth and the maintenance of skeletal integrity [38].

Taurine transporters are present in bone-forming cells, specifically osteoblasts, where they play a crucial role in maintaining bone homeostasis. Taurine promotes the development of osteoblasts, and its supplementation activates the extracellular signal-regulated kinase (ERK) pathway, leading to increased osteoblast activity. By enhancing the activity of alkaline phosphatase (ALP), a key marker of osteoblast differentiation, taurine supports bone formation and facilitates bone mineralization in a concentration-dependent manner. Furthermore, taurine stimulates the production of osteogenic growth factors, which further aid osteoblast function. Beyond fostering bone formation, taurine also helps prevent bone loss by suppressing osteoclast activity and reducing bone resorption.

One proposed mechanism involves the regulation of the Na^+/Ca^{2+} exchanger (NCX). Under normal conditions, NCX exports Ca^{2+} from cells in exchange for Na^+. In its reverse mode, however, NCX imports Ca^{2+} and exports Na^+, leading to intracellular calcium overload that disrupts the function of bone cells. NCX is localized on the mineralizing surface of osteoblasts, where it plays a crucial role in calcium homeostasis.

In their 2021 study, Berry and colleagues propose that bone mineral density in osteoporotic patients may be enhanced *via* a four-nutraceutical supplementation strategy (taurine, calcium, vitamin D and vitamin K). This strategy could potentially decrease the disability and mortality linked to fragility fractures, though robust clinical evidence remains required [1].

7.2 Vitamin D and osteoporosis

In the United States, adults aged 51 to 70 years are advised to take a vitamin D supplement of 400 IU, while those over 70 years should take 600 IU. Conversely, the European Commission recommends a daily intake of 400 IU for individuals aged 65 years and older. The maximum acceptable daily intake of vitamin D is set at 2000 IU.

The level at which no adverse effects are observed is estimated to be 10,000 IU per day, while the lowest level at which adverse effects may occur is 40,000 IU per day. Although the exact threshold for vitamin D toxicity is not precisely defined, it is expected to be significantly higher than these doses. However, high-dose supplementation can lead to hypercalcemia, which may impair kidney function.

Factors that increase the risk of vitamin D toxicity include excessive calcium intake, existing hypercalcemia, idiopathic hypercalciuria, sarcoidosis, overproduction of vitamin D metabolites, reduced vitamin D binding, and hypersensitivity to vitamin D.

For postmenopausal women, the need for vitamin D and calcium supplementation is not considered essential, and significant caution is not required [39, 40].

Nevertheless, studies have shown that the lower levels of 25(OH)D are associated with a higher incidence of albuminuria, which is a known risk factor for the progression of chronic kidney disease. Cigarette smoking is a significant risk factor for Osteoporosis. Within the tar fraction of cigarette smoke, about 4700 chemical constituents have been identified, with nicotine being the only compound consistently linked to negative effects on bone remodelling. Nicotine inhibits the activity and proliferation of osteoblasts while promoting the differentiation and resorptive activity of osteoclasts. Additionally, nicotine induces oxidative stress, as demonstrated in numerous *in vitro* and *in vivo* studies. It activates the NF-κB signalling pathway, indirectly contributing to osteoclastogenesis and increasing pro-inflammatory cytokines, such as IL-1 and IL-6, in animal models [39–41].

Vitamin E supplementation has been studied as a protective measure against nicotine-induced bone loss. Tocotrienols, which are powerful lipid-soluble antioxidants, have been shown to suppress nicotine-induced increases in pro-inflammatory cytokines IL-1 and IL-6 at high doses. In contrast, tocopherols do not significantly affect these cytokines. Therefore, among the two main forms of vitamin E examined, tocotrienols appear to be more effective than tocopherols in reducing bone resorption by modulating inflammatory mediators and decreasing bone loss [40].

7.3 Zinc

Zinc plays a crucial anabolic role in bone metabolism, with bone tissue acting as a reservoir for this mineral. During the process of bone resorption, zinc is released and later reincorporated into the bone matrix. Research indicates that the calcium-to-zinc ratio in the vertebrae declines with age in humans, suggesting that zinc is conserved more than calcium as individuals grow older.

Zinc is incorporated into the mineral component of hydroxyapatite and may form complexes with fluoride; both zinc and the zinc-fluoride complex are believed to enhance the crystallinity of apatite. In individuals with Osteoporosis, skeletal zinc levels are typically reduced. Zinc is recognized as a biomarker for bone resorption.

Several studies have shown that postmenopausal women tend to have elevated urinary zinc excretion, with those suffering from Osteoporosis excreting more than 800 μg per gram of creatinine in their urine.

Supplementation with trace minerals, either alone or in combination with calcium, has been demonstrated to improve bone mineral density in postmenopausal women. Research conducted in both *in vitro* (test tube) and *in vivo* (living organism) settings supports the positive effects of zinc on bone metabolism. For example, administering zinc sulphate (5 or 10 mg of zinc per kg of body weight) to weanling rats for 3 days resulted in a dose-dependent increase in zinc levels, DNA, collagen, calcium and alkaline phosphatase activity in the femoral diaphysis (the main shaft of the thigh bone).

Alkaline phosphatase activity in osteoblasts (bone-building cells) is associated with bone mineralization, and osteoblasts are also responsible for producing collagen, which is an essential protein for bone structure. The DNA content in bone tissue reflects the number of bone cells present, including osteoblasts, osteoclasts, and osteocytes. Therefore, the accumulation of zinc in bone is beneficial, as it enhances alkaline phosphatase activity and stimulates collagen production in osteoblasts, indirectly supporting bone mineralization and calcification [35, 40–42].

7.4 Curcumin

Curcumin plays a significant role in modulating bone remodelling by inhibiting osteoclastogenesis. It specifically suppresses the differentiation of osteoclast precursors into mature osteoclasts by downregulating the chemokine CCL3. Additionally, it hinders the expression of critical osteoclast differentiation markers—cathepsin K, MMP-9 and MMP-13—by upregulating miR-365. Moreover, curcumin demonstrates immunomodulatory effects on macrophages, attenuating inflammatory responses, reducing the release of proinflammatory mediators and limiting osteoclast formation. Collectively, these effects are mediated, at least in part, through the modulation of the Akt/NF-κB/NFATc1 signalling pathway.

7.5 Alliaceae and Brassicaceae

Edible plants from the Allium and Brassica families (Alliaceae and Brassicaceae) contain organic sulphur compounds (OSCs) that have been shown to enhance both the proliferation and viability of mesenchymal stem cells (MSCs), while simultaneously suppressing these processes in monocytes. Furthermore, these compounds facilitate osteogenic differentiation and promote bone formation, inhibiting osteoclast differentiation at various stages. This dual mechanism helps minimize bone erosion and reduces the viability of osteocytes. Notably, compounds such as allicin, allyl sulphide, sulphoraphane and glucoraphanin are recognized for their critical roles in regulating bone metabolism. Polysulphides found in the Alliaceae family, along with glucosinolates and isothiocyanates from the Brassicaceae family, exhibit anti-inflammatory, antioxidant, vasorelaxant and hypolipidemic properties. These bioactive compounds stimulate osteoblast activity while inhibiting osteoclast activity by releasing hydrogen sulphide, which functions as a gasotransmitter [41].

Onions (*Allium cepa* L.) are rich in flavonoids and organosulphur compounds that promote bone health by reducing bone resorption and enhancing bone mineral density (BMD) in women during and after menopause. Similarly, garlic (*Allium sativum*), when taken in tablet form for 30 days, has been shown to lower oxidative stress in menopausal women, potentially helping to delay the onset and progression of Osteoporosis. Additionally, both garlic and leeks possess properties that inhibit bone resorption.

Probiotics are beneficial microorganisms that play a crucial role in the gastrointestinal microbiota. Common probiotic species include *Lactobacillus*, *Bifidobacterium*, *Escherichia coli*, *Enterococcus*, *Bacillus subtilis* and several species of *Saccharomyces*. Increasing evidence suggests that these microorganisms can influence bone metabolism by acting on the RANKL/RANK/OPG pathway, thereby supporting bone formation and reducing bone loss, particularly under conditions of oestrogen deficiency.

Experimental studies have shown that supplementation with *Lactobacillus reuteri* can prevent osteoporosis associated with type 1 diabetes. This effect appears to occur through inhibition of tumour necrosis factor (TNF)-mediated suppression of Wnt10b signalling. Similar benefits have been observed in glucocorticoid-induced osteoporosis, where *L. reuteri* supplementation has been reported to improve bone density by restoring Wnt10b activity and modulating osteoclast function. Wnt10b plays a key role in bone formation by promoting osteoblast differentiation, partly through the downregulation of peroxisome proliferator-activated receptor gamma (PPAR-γ) [35, 42].

7.6 Prebiotics

Prebiotics act differently. They are not digested directly but are fermented by gut bacteria to produce short-chain fatty acids (SCFAs), such as acetate, propionate and butyrate. These metabolites have been shown to improve the absorption of minerals, including calcium and magnesium, in both animal and human studies. One proposed explanation is that SCFAs lower caecal pH, which enhances mineral solubility and absorption. Over time, this process may contribute to an improvement in bone mineral density [42].

7.7 Postbiotics

Postbiotics are bioactive substances that are produced during the fermentation of foods by food-grade microorganisms. Unlike probiotics, these compounds are not live organisms. Instead, they encompass a broad range of microbial products, including metabolites, short-chain fatty acids (SCFAs), fragments of microbial cells, functional proteins, extracellular polymeric substances (EPSs), cell lysates, teichoic acids, peptidoglycan-derived muropeptides and pili-like structures. These components are believed to exert their health effects primarily through their interaction with the gut microbiota.

Although research on postbiotics is still relatively new, recent studies suggest that they play a role in bone health. In ovariectomized (OVX) rat models, postbiotics obtained from *Bacillus coagulans* were reported to improve bone mineral density (BMD). Similar findings have been observed in experimental models of postmenopausal osteoporosis. In a mouse model, the postbiotic *Lactobacillus curvatus* 38-CS was shown to reduce bone loss by inhibiting RANKL-induced osteoclast differentiation. This effect was associated with suppression of the TRAF6/NF-κB/MAPK signalling pathway, which is known to be involved in osteoclast activation.

7.8 Synbiotics

Synbiotics are formulations that blend probiotics and prebiotics, which work together synergistically to enhance their individual contributions to bone health. In studies involving ovariectomized (OVX) rats, supplementation with a mixture of fructooligosaccharides (FOS) and soy isoflavones led to improvements in trabecular bone microarchitecture. Furthermore, when FOS was paired with dried plum fractions in soy-based diets, researchers observed a more significant increase in whole-body bone mineral density (BMD). Additional investigations revealed that administering FOS alongside *Bifidobacterium longum* resulted in enhanced calcium (Ca), magnesium (Mg) and phosphorus (P) content in bones, as well as improved bone-breaking strength in rats. Similarly, the combination of *Bifidobacterium longum* with galactooligosaccharides (GOS) increased the bioavailability of Ca, Mg and P, along with boosting the bone mineral content in the hind limbs [35, 42].

7.9 Melatonin

Melatonin (N-acetyl-5-methoxytryptamine) is a bioamine predominantly secreted by the pineal gland during the nocturnal phase. While its primary role involves regulating circadian rhythms, melatonin exerts multifaceted influences on various physiological processes, including thermoregulation, reproductive function, immune response, cardiovascular regulation, energy metabolism and bone physiology. These effects are primarily mediated *via* melatonin receptor 2 (MT2R), which is expressed on mesenchymal stem cells (MSCs), osteoblasts and osteoclasts. Recent investigations have increasingly underscored the anti-osteoporotic potential of melatonin. Dysregulated melatonin levels have been implicated in the pathogenesis and progression of Osteoporosis, with particular relevance to postmenopausal women. Mechanistically, melatonin promotes osteoblast proliferation and differentiation, facilitates the synthesis and mineralization of extracellular matrix (ECM), and enhances cortical bone formation. Experimental studies in Wistar rats have demonstrated that melatonin supplementation results in significant improvements in bone mass, volume and mechanical stiffness, thereby enhancing skeletal integrity compared to untreated controls. These findings suggest that melatonin misa promising therapeutic agent for the prevention and management of Osteoporosis [39–41].

Consequently, melatonin (Mel) enhances osteoblast formation while simultaneously inhibiting the production of osteoclasts and adipocytes. In rat models, Mel has been shown to counteract the decline in osteogenic differentiation capacity of bone marrow mesenchymal stem cells (MSCs)—a decline often associated with Osteoporosis. Furthermore, it reverses the detrimental effects of tumour necrosis factor (TNF) on osteogenic differentiation and inflammation in bone marrow stem cells (BMSCs) by inhibiting NF-κB signalling pathways.

In ovariectomized (OVX) mice, Mel promotes osteogenic differentiation of BMSCs and prevents bone loss through the HGF/PTEN/Wnt/β-catenin axis. Specifically, hepatocyte growth factor (HGF) downregulates PTEN, leading to activation of the Wnt/β-catenin pathway both *in vitro* and *in vivo* [42].

In OVX rats with tibial defects as a model of Osteoporosis, Mel has been shown to facilitate the coupling of osteogenesis and angiogenesis mediated by BMSCs. It stimulates angiogenesis by upregulating vascular endothelial growth factor (VEGF) and increases the expression of key markers associated with bone formation and vascularization, compared with untreated controls [39].

Melatonin also exerts a potent anti-resorptive effect by modulating osteoblast and osteoclast interactions:

It suppresses RANKL (a pro-osteoclastogenic factor) while upregulating osteoprotegerin (OPG), the natural inhibitor of RANKL.

It thereby antagonizes osteoclast differentiation and function.

Additionally, Mel inhibits the SIRT signalling pathway, which would otherwise suppress NF-κB signalling and promote osteoclastogenesis.

Beyond this, Mel inhibits the osteoclastogenic differentiation of haematopoietic stem cells and protects bone marrow cells from the cytotoxic effects of the chemotherapeutic agent aracytin. However, the specific cellular source of melatonin within the bone marrow microenvironment remains to be fully identified [40].

In a rat model of Osteoporosis induced by glucocorticoids, it was observed that high doses of dexamethasone trigger ferroptosis in bone marrow stem cells (BMSCs)—a type of programmed cell death that relies on iron. The early introduction of melatonin (Mel) was found to block this ferroptotic pathway, underscoring its potential for osteoporosis prevention. This protective mechanism operates by inhibiting the PI3K/AKT/mTOR signalling pathway, which is crucial for regulating bone metabolism [41].

In a mouse model of type 2 diabetes with Osteoporosis, the elevated glucose levels were found to trigger ferroptosis through the increase of reactive oxygen species (ROS), lipid peroxidation and depletion of glutathione. Mel treatment mitigated this effect by stimulating the nuclear factor erythroid 2-related factor 2 (Nrf2)/haeme oxygenase-1 (HO-1) pathway. This activation enhanced the osteogenic potential of osteoblasts, a finding further validated *in vitro* [42].

In osteoclasts, Mel exerts an inhibitory effect on both differentiation and function by reducing RANKL-induced ROS production through suppression of NF-κB signalling. This not only mitigates oxidative stress and inflammation but also protects osteoblasts, thereby preventing ROS- and cytokine-driven osteolysis.

Mitochondria, as the main generators of free radicals and oxidative stress, play a pivotal role in ageing-related diseases such as Osteoporosis. Mitochondrial dysfunction impairs osteogenesis while simultaneously enhancing osteoclastic activity, thereby accelerating bone loss. Importantly, Mel functions as an endogenous mitochondria-targeted antioxidant, reducing oxidative stress within bone cells and protecting against age-related skeletal deterioration.

7.10 Fatty acids and bone health

The intake and plasma levels of fatty acids impact bone health in different ways depending on the number of double bonds in their carbon chains. Diets high in saturated fatty acids (SFAs), particularly high-fat diets, are generally harmful to bone health. Several mechanisms contribute to this negative effect: 1. Formation of complexes with calcium and other minerals in the gut, leading to their excretion in faeces. 2. Altered synthesis of prostaglandins. 3. Impaired osteoblast differentiation and activity. 4. Increased lipid oxidation. Palmitic acid, which is one of the most abundant SFAs in the human diet, is particularly detrimental as it induces apoptosis in osteoblasts while promoting the survival of osteoclasts by preventing their programmed cell death.

Numerous studies have shown a positive association between total lipid intake and fracture risk, as well as an inverse relationship between lipid intake and bone mineral density (BMD). In contrast, polyunsaturated fatty acids (PUFAs) offer protective effects on bone, particularly in terms of fracture prevention. Omega-3 fatty acids play a crucial role by regulating osteoblast and osteoclast activity, modulating inflammatory responses, and influencing calcium metabolism. The role of omega-6 fatty acids, however, remains less established.

Overall, higher total PUFA intake has been associated with increased BMD and a reduced risk of fractures. Omega-3 fatty acids protect against bone loss through three main mechanisms: 1. Enhancing intestinal calcium absorption. 2. Suppressing the activity of inflammatory cytokines. 3. Modulating peroxisome proliferator-activated receptor (PPAR) activity, which affects bone remodelling. The composition of dietary fat has a significant influence on calcium absorption and urinary calcium levels. PUFAs enhance intestinal calcium uptake by increasing the activity of Ca^{2+}-ATPase, a key enzyme in active calcium transport.

Dietary sources of omega-3 fatty acids include alpha-linolenic acid (ALA), primarily obtained from foods such as walnuts, flaxseeds, chia seeds and vegetable oils like soy and flaxseed oil. Eicosapentaenoic acid (EPA) and docosahexaenoic acid (DHA) are predominantly found in fatty fish. Epidemiological evidence supports these mechanistic findings. For instance, in a study involving 891 menopausal women, dietary intake was evaluated using a Food Frequency Questionnaire (FFQ), and BMD was measured *via* dual-energy X-ray absorptiometry (DEXA). The results indicated a negative association between high fatty acid intake and loss of femoral BMD. Moreover, a higher ratio of omega-6 to omega-3 fatty acids was linked to lower BMD at the hip in both men and women [35, 43].

7.11 Green tea and bone health

In recent decades, there has been a growing interest in the potential connection between green tea consumption, bone mineral density (BMD) and Osteoporosis. Green tea is rich in several bioactive compounds that are beneficial for bone health. Its polyphenols exhibit antioxidant properties, which help protect osteoblasts from oxidative stress, thereby aiding in the maintenance of BMD. Moreover, green tea contains isoflavones, which possesses mild estrogenic activity and may help reduce bone resorption, particularly in postmenopausal women. While some studies find no significant association between green tea intake and BMD, a substantial body of evidence supports a positive correlation. Two meta-analyses of observational studies have concluded that tea consumption is linked to higher BMD and a decreased risk of Osteoporosis. However, these benefits seem to diminish with excessive tea consumption—specifically, more than approximately five cups per day—primarily due to the effects of caffeine. Caffeine may counteract the bone-protective effects of polyphenols and isoflavones through several mechanisms. First, as a purine-like compound, it antagonizes adenosine by competitively inhibiting A2 receptors, which suppresses bone formation while promoting resorption. Additionally, caffeine affects calcium metabolism by increasing urinary calcium excretion and interfering with the activity of vitamin D receptors. Taken together, these mechanisms indicate that while moderate green tea consumption may be advantageous for bone health, excessive intake could pose risks [34].

7.12 Phytoestrogens and bone health

Phytoestrogens are non-steroidal, naturally occurring polyphenolic compounds that structurally resemble endogenous oestrogens. They can be broadly classified into isoflavones, stilbenes, coumestans and lignans, with isoflavones, which are abundant in soy and other legumes, being the most extensively studied. The development of postmenopausal Osteoporosis is primarily driven by oestrogen deficiency, leading to unchecked osteoclast activity during bone resorption. Although phytoestrogens bind to oestrogen receptors with a lower affinity than endogenous hormones, they elicit similar protective effects. Their antioxidant properties further enhance their potential role in promoting bone health.

Evidence from animal models and *in vitro* studies suggests that phytoestrogens can mitigate bone mineral density (BMD) loss by simultaneously inhibiting resorption and promoting bone formation. Although human data is more limited, the results are encouraging. Systematic reviews and meta-analyses of randomized controlled trials indicate that isoflavones contribute to maintaining BMD and decreasing bone resorption in both pre- and postmenopausal women. For instance, a study by Somekawa et al. found that soy isoflavones slowed bone loss in the lumbar spine of perimenopausal women. Additionally, glabrene, an isoflavone found in liquorice root, has been identified as a potential therapeutic agent in this regard. Among other phytoestrogens, resveratrol, a stilbene present in grape skins and red berries, has shown promise in clinical studies by improving BMD in the femoral neck and lumbar spine of postmenopausal women. While further well-designed clinical trials are necessary to ascertain efficacy and safety, phytoestrogens represent a cost-effective and natural complementary strategy for the prevention and treatment of postmenopausal Osteoporosis [36, 37].

7.13 Phytoestrogens and flavonoids in bone health

Phytoestrogens exert their biological effects primarily by binding to oestrogen receptors α (ERα) and β (ERβ), with many phytoestrogens showing a higher affinity for ERβ. Due to their structural similarity to 17β-estradiol, phytoestrogens act as selective oestrogen receptor modulators (SERMs). Although they mimic the effects of estradiol, their activity is significantly weaker—approximately 1 to 0.1% of that of endogenous oestrogen. Among the dietary bioactive compounds, flavonoids found in fruits, vegetables, herbs, spices, essential oils and beverages show the most promise in supporting bone health. They influence bone remodelling by modulating cellular signalling pathways that regulate the differentiation of osteoblasts and osteoclasts, thereby promoting bone formation while inhibiting resorption [36, 37, 39].

One notable example is Equol (7-hydroxy-3-(4′-hydroxyphenyl)chroman), an isoflavone produced through gut bacterial metabolism of the soy isoflavone daidzein. Equol has a strong affinity for ERβ and plays a role in bone protection. In osteoclast progenitor cells, receptor activator of nuclear factor-κB ligand (RANKL) and reactive oxygen species (ROS) stimulate the expression of tumour necrosis factor-alpha (TNF-α), which in turn enhances bone resorption. Rutin, a flavonol glycoside, counteracts this process by reducing ROS generation and suppressing TNF-α expression, thus inhibiting osteoclast formation. Other flavonoids also demonstrate the potent effects on skeletal health [37].

Monomeric flavanols—including catechin, epicatechin, gallocatechin, epigallocatechin and epigallocatechin gallate from *Camellia sinensis* leaves—can increase serum levels of bone-specific alkaline phosphatase, a biomarker for bone formation. Similarly, grape seed proanthocyanidins have been shown to enhance both bone formation and strength. The citrus flavanone hesperidin has shown protective effects against Osteoporosis in both men and women by slowing down bone resorption and regulating inflammatory mediators. Olive polyphenols, such as oleuropein, oleocanthin, tyrosol and hydroxytyrosol, stimulate osteoblast activity while inhibiting osteoclastogenesis. Resveratrol (3,5,4′-trihydroxystilbene), a stilbene found in grapes, peanuts and wine, acts as a potent antioxidant and binds to both oestrogen receptors (ERα and ERβ). Its various actions on osteoblasts and osteoclasts give it the potential to reduce bone resorption and contribute to skeletal protection [36, 37].

7.14 Essential oils, antioxidant vitamins and bone health

Essential oils such as thyme, sage, rosemary, juniper, pine, mountain pine, turpentine and eucalyptus, along with their monoterpene components (including thujone, eucalyptol, camphor, borneol, thymol, α-pinene, β-pinene, bornyl acetate, and menthol), have been shown to inhibit bone resorption. Specifically, pine oil protects against bone loss, while the monoterpenes borneol, thymol and camphor exert a direct inhibitory effect on osteoclast activity. Additionally, verbenol, a metabolite of α-pinene, has been shown to possess osteoclast-suppressing properties. Recent clinical evidence supports the role of antioxidant vitamins in bone health. In a study involving 75 osteoporotic patients, supplementation with vitamin E (400 mg) and vitamin C (500 mg) for 90 days enhanced bone mineral density (BMD) and reduced the levels of inflammatory markers, highlighting the antioxidant-mediated protective effect against Osteoporosis [31].

7.15 Potassium and bone metabolism

Potassium plays a crucial role in maintaining calcium homeostasis, particularly by regulating the conservation and excretion of urinary calcium. Diets low in potassium lead to increased urinary calcium loss, whereas potassium-rich diets help mitigate this issue. Abundant in fruits, vegetables, legumes and dairy products, potassium is known for its alkaline ash properties, which counterbalance the acid load associated with typical Western diets. Research has shown a correlation between net endogenous acid production (NEAP), potassium intake and bone mineral density (BMD), underscoring the importance of potassium for maintaining skeletal health. Potassium citrate supplementation has been shown to reduce bone resorption, which is often triggered by high salt intake. Furthermore, higher potassium consumption—particularly from fruits and vegetables—has been associated with a higher baseline BMD and a lower rate of bone loss over time. These findings support public health recommendations to consume five to ten servings of fruits and vegetables daily, promoting bone health.

7.16 Vitamin K and bone health

Vitamin K is a fat-soluble vitamin that plays a crucial role in blood clotting and bone health. It acts as a cofactor for enzymes that facilitate the carboxylation of osteocalcin, a protein essential for bone mineralization. Additionally, vitamin K helps to reduce urinary calcium loss, contributing to stronger bones. Rich dietary sources of vitamin K include dark green leafy vegetables, fruits and vegetable oils, while smaller amounts can be found in dairy products and grains. Vitamin K_2, a specific form of vitamin K, is particularly abundant in fermented dairy and soy products, as well as in fish, meat, liver and eggs. The recommended adequate intake (AI) is 120 micrograms (μg) per day for men and 90 μg per day for women. Observational studies have shown a positive correlation between vitamin K intake and serum levels, leading to increased bone density. Moreover, individuals who experience fractures often have lower serum levels of vitamin K. Epidemiological research suggests that a higher intake of vitamin K is linked to a reduced risk of fractures. A high proportion of undercarboxylated serum osteocalcin, typically observed in individuals with low serum vitamin K levels, may indicate a higher risk of fractures. However, many studies examining this relationship are complicated by overall poor nutrition. In contrast, research involving healthy girls consuming a typical US diet has shown that improved vitamin K status is associated with reduced bone turnover.

Vitamin K deficiency or antagonism—particularly due to coumarin derivatives—can lead to undercarboxylation of key proteins involved in bone metabolism, such as osteocalcin. Cohort studies have identified that using warfarin for over a year is an independent predictor of spine and hip fractures. However, this association was not confirmed in another study, possibly due to the limited number of women on warfarin in that sample. Several small controlled studies on vitamin K supplementation have reported reductions in calcium excretion, bone resorption and the undercarboxylated fraction of osteocalcin. A compound derived from vitamin K, known as MK4, has shown a positive effect on bone mineral density (BMD) in high doses when administered to women with Osteoporosis and strokes.

Additionally, high pharmacologic doses of vitamin K_2 (45 mg) were associated with the lower rates of bone loss and a reduced incidence of fractures. Despite existing evidence from observational studies, research on intermediate endpoints, and small studies examining bone density and limited fracture data, there is still insufficient information to recommend a specific level of vitamin K supplementation for optimal bone health. One trial involving a three-year supplementation of phylloquinone (1 mg/day) combined with calcium and vitamin D successfully reduced hip bone loss. Generally, a healthy diet rich in fruits and vegetables provides adequate vitamin K intake for most of the population.

7.17 Magnesium and bone health

Magnesium, when bound to adenosine triphosphate (ATP), plays a crucial role in numerous enzymatic reactions, particularly those involved in protein and nucleic acid synthesis. Approximately 60% of the body's total magnesium is stored in bones, where it plays a crucial role in mineralization and regulates the activity of both osteoblasts and osteoclasts. The recommended dietary allowance (RDA) is 420 mg per day for men and 320 mg per day for women. Despite its abundant presence in legumes, vegetables, nuts, seeds, fruits, grains, fish and dairy products, many individuals—especially in the United States—consume magnesium at levels below the recommended amounts. Insufficient magnesium intake has been linked to decreased bone mineral density (BMD), Osteoporosis and an increased risk of fractures. Supplementation with magnesium may be particularly advantageous for frail elderly individuals with subpar diets, those suffering from intestinal disorders, alcohol dependence or patients undergoing diuretic or chemotherapy treatment, as these conditions can lead to magnesium depletion. Additionally, since calcium supplementation is sometimes associated with constipation, magnesium supplementation may provide gastrointestinal benefits by promoting regular bowel movements. Magnesium deficiency can be identified through biochemical markers, including reduced serum magnesium and calcium levels, as well as resistance to vitamin D.

Clinical manifestations of deficiency may include muscle twitching, cramps, hypertension and cardiac arrhythmias. Fortunately, magnesium deficiency is treatable. Several small epidemiological studies suggest that higher magnesium intake is associated with increased BMD in older men and women. However, relatively few controlled clinical trials have examined magnesium supplementation, and most positive findings have been observed in individuals with pre-existing magnesium deficiency. Currently, the evidence regarding the role of magnesium in preventing Osteoporosis in the general population remains inconclusive. Data from the Women's Health Initiative (WHI) indicated that higher intakes of magnesium may be associated with an increased risk of wrist fractures, suggesting that excessive supplementation may not be beneficial for everyone.

7.18 Herba Epimedii

Icaridin, a component of the traditional Chinese medication Herba Epimedii, can prevent inflammatory bone loss by inhibiting osteoclastogenesis induced by lipopolysaccharide, TNF-α, and IL-6, while promoting type-2 cyclooxygenase and prostaglandin E2 production.

8. Conclusion

Osteoporosis is a silent, age-related disorder influenced by a variety of factors. It can be prevented through lifestyle modifications and a balanced diet, as nutraceuticals offer numerous beneficial properties. Several studies, both animal and human, have highlighted the positive impact of these compounds on maintaining bone microstructure; however, further research involving human subjects is necessary to confirm these findings. Nutraceuticals, including specific vitamins and minerals, promote osteoblastogenesis while suppressing oxidative stress markers and apoptotic signals.

Author details

Shah Waliullah[1], Zeenat Ara[1], Ankit Sriwastava[1], Vivek Kumar Verma[1], Anand Kumar[1], Devarshi Rastogi[1], Shatakshi Pant[1], Virendra Pandey[1], Uday Raj[1] and Ram Lakhan Singh[2*]

1 Department of Orthopaedic Surgery, King George's Medical University, Chowk, Lucknow, Uttar Pradesh, India

2 Department of Biochemistry, Dr. Ram Manohar Lohia Avadh University, Faizabad, India

*Address all correspondence to: drrlsingh123@gmail.com

References

[1] Ara Z, Pandey S, Pant S, Tripathi RM, Rastogi D, Waliullah S. Osteoporosis, its pathophysiology and effect of nutraceuticals. Indian Journal of Public Health Research & Development. 2023;**14**(3):385-391

[2] Chadha M, Chaddha R, Divakar H, Kalyan H, Seth S, Shah P. Osteoporosis: Epidemiology, pathogenesis, evaluation and treatment. Open Journal of Orthopedics. 2022;**12**(4):153-182

[3] de Villiers TJ, Goldstein SR. Bone health 2022: An update. Climacteric. 2022;**25**(1):1-3. DOI: 10.1080/13697137.2021.1965408

[4] Panday K, Gona A, Humphrey MB. Medication-induced osteoporosis: Screening and treatment strategies. Therapeutic Advances in Musculoskeletal Disease. 2014;**6**:185-202

[5] Dobbs MB, Buckwalter J, Saltzman C. Osteoporosis: The increasing role of the orthopaedist. The Iowa Orthopaedic Journal. 1999;**19**:43-52. Available from: http://www.ncbi.nlm.nih.gov/pubmed/10847516

[6] Arron JR, Choi Y. Bone versus immune system. Nature. 2000;**408**(6812):535-536. DOI: 10.1038/35046196

[7] Hanley DA, Adachi JD, Bell A, Brown V. Denosumab: Mechanism of action and clinical outcomes. International Journal of Clinical Practice. 2012;**66**:1139-1146

[8] Leder BZ, Tsai JN, Uihlein AV, Wallace PM, Lee H, Neer RM, et al. Denosumab and teriparatide transitions in postmenopausal osteoporosis (the DATA-switch study): Extension of a randomized controlled trial. The Lancet. 2015;**386**(9999):1147-1155

[9] Abrahamsen B, van Staa T, Ariely R, Olson M, Cooper C. Excess mortality following hip fracture: A systematic epidemiological review. Osteoporosis International. 2009;**20**(10):1633-1650

[10] Colón-Emeric C, Kuchibhatla M, Pieper C, et al. The contribution of hip fracture to risk of subsequent fractures: Data from two longitudinal studies. Osteoporosis International. 2003;**11**:879-883

[11] Office of the Surgeon General (US). Bone Health and Osteoporosis: A Report of the Surgeon General. Rockville (MD): Office of the Surgeon General (US); 2004. Available from: http://www.ncbi.nlm.nih.gov/books/NBK45513/ [Accessed: March, 2014]

[12] Lewiecki EM, Laster AJ. Clinical review: Clinical applications of vertebral fracture assessment by dual-energy x-ray absorptiometry. The Journal of Clinical Endocrinology and Metabolism. 2006;**91**(11):4215-4222

[13] Riggs BL, Melton LJ III. Evidence for two distinct syndromes of involutional osteoporosis. The American Journal of Medicine. 1983;**75**:899-901

[14] Riggs BL, Khosla S, Melton LJ III. A unitary model for involutional osteoporosis: Estrogen deficiency causes both type I and type II osteoporosis in postmenopausal women and contributes to bone loss in aging men. Journal of Bone and Mineral Research. 1998;**13**:763-773

[15] Delitala AP, Scuteri A, Doria C. Thyroid hormone diseases and

osteoporosis. Journal of Clinical Medicine. 2020;**9**:1034. DOI: 10.3390/jcm9041034

[16] Kanis JA, Cooper C, Rizzoli R, et al. Executive summary of European guidance for the diagnosis and management of osteoporosis in postmenopausal women. Aging Clinical and Experimental Research. 2019;**31**:15-17

[17] Kanis JA, Harvey NC, Johansson H, et al. A decade of FRAX: How has it changed the management of osteoporosis? Aging Clinical and Experimental Research. 2020;**32**:187-196

[18] Kanis JA, Harvey NC, McCloskey E, et al. Algorithm for the management of patients at low/middle/high risk of osteoporotic fracture: A global perspective. Osteoporosis International. 2020;**31**:1-12. DOI: 10.1007/s00198-019-05176-3

[19] Cosman F, Nieves JW, Dempster DW. Treatment sequence matters: Anabolic and antiresorptive therapy for osteoporosis. Journal of Bone and Mineral Research. 2017;**32**:198-202

[20] Kendler DL, Marin F, Zerbini CAF, et al. Efects of teriparatide and risedronate on new fractures in postmenopausal women with severe osteoporosis (VERO): A multicentre, double-blind, double-dummy, randomized controlled trial. Lancet. 2018;**391**:230-240 (Erratum Lancet 2018; 392: 2352)

[21] Saag KG, Petersen J, Brandi ML, et al. Romosozumab or alendronate for fracture prevention in women with osteoporosis. The New England Journal of Medicine. 2017;**377**:1417-1427

[22] National Institute for Health and Care Excellence (NICE). Bisphosphonates for treating osteoporosis. In: Technology Appraisal Guidance. Vol. 464. London: National Institute for Health and Care Excellence; 2017

[23] Kanis JA, Rizzoli R, Cooper C, et al. Challenges for the development of bone forming agents in Europe. Calcified Tissue International. 2014;**94**:469-473

[24] Leder BZ, Tsai JN, Neer RM, et al. Response to therapy with teriparatide, denosumab, or both in postmenopausal women in the DATA (Denosumab and Teriparatide administration) study randomized controlled trial. Journal of Clinical Densitometry. 2016;**19**:346-351

[25] Inque M, Tanaka H, Moriwake T, Oka M, Sekiguchi C, Seino Y. Altered biochemical markers of bone turnover in humans during 120 days of bed rest. Bone. 2000;**26**(3):281-286

[26] Veitch SW, Findlay SC, Hamer AJ, Blumsohn A, Eastell R, Ingle BM. Changes in bone mass and bone turnover following tibial shaft fracture. Osteoporosis International. 2006;**17**:364-372

[27] Hannon R, Eastell R. Preanalytical variability of biochemical markers of bone turnover. Osteoporosis International. 2000;**11**(Suppl. 6): S30-S44

[28] Parker SE, Troisi R, Wise LA, Palmer JR, Titus-Ernstoff L, Strohsnitter WC, et al. Menarche, menopause, years of menstruation, and the incidence of osteoporosis: The influence of prenatal exposure to diethylstilbestrol. The Journal of Clinical Endocrinology & Metabolism. 2014;**99**(2):594-601

[29] Mitra S, Desai M, Khatkhatay MI. Vitamin D receptor gene polymorphisms

and bone mineral density in postmenopausal Indian women. Maturitas. 2006;**55**(1):27-35

[30] Bischoff-Ferrari HA, Willett WC, Wong JB, Stuck AE, Staehelin HB, Orav EJ, et al. Prevention of nonvertebral fractures with oral vitamin D and dose dependency: A meta-analysis of randomized controlled trials. Archives of Internal Medicine. 2009;**169**:551-561

[31] Bouillon R, Marcocci C, Carmeliet G, Bikle D, White JH, Dawson-Hughes B, et al. Skeletal and extraskeletal actions of vitamin D: Current evidence and outstanding questions. Endocrine Reviews. 2019;**40**:1109-1151

[32] Nakamura K, Saito T, Oyama M, et al. Vitamin D sufficiency is associated with low incidence of limb and vertebral fractures in community-dwelling elderly Japanese women: The Muramatsu study. Osteoporosis International. 2011;**22**:97-103. DOI: 10.1007/s00198-010-1213-6

[33] Pietschmann P, Mechtcheriakova D, Meshcheryakova A, Föger-Samwald U, Ellinger I. Immunology of osteoporosis: A mini-review. Gerontology. 2016;**62**(2):128-137

[34] European Commission. Report on Osteoporosis in the European Community — Action for Prevention. Luxembourg: Office for Official Publications of the European Communities; 1998

[35] Yamaguchi M. Role of nutritional zinc in the prevention of osteoporosis. Molecular and Cellular Biochemistry. 2010;**338**(1):241-254

[36] Vieth E. Vitamin D supplementation, 25-hydroxyvitamin D concentrations, and safety. The American Journal of Clinical Nutrition. 1999;**69**:842-856

[37] Taylor RL, Lynch HJ, Wysor WG. Seasonal influence of sunlight on the hypercalcemia of sarcoidosis. The American Journal of Medicine. 1963;**34**:221-227

[38] Srivastava RN, Ara Z, Waliullah S, Singh A, Raj S, Mahdi AA, et al. Taurine is a future biomolecule for potential health benefits: A review. Journal of Metabolomics and Systems Biology. 2022;**5**(1):1-3

[39] Florence S, Baker R, Adrizzo JR, et al. Hyperalcaemia in mycobacterial infection. The Journal of Clinical Endocrinology. 1972;**34**:251-256

[40] Haussler MR, McCain TA. Basic and clinical concepts related to vitamin D metabolism and action. The New England Journal of Medicine. 1977;**297**:1041-1050

[41] de Boer IH, Ioannou GN, Kestenbaum B, Brunzell JD, Weiss NS. 25-hydroxyvitamin D levels and albuminuria in the third National Health and Nutrition Examination Survey (NHANES III). American Journal of Kidney Diseases. 2007;**50**:69-77

[42] Nazrun AS, Norazlina M, Norliza M, Nirwana SI. The anti-inflammatory role of vitamin E in prevention of osteoporosis. Advances in Pharmacological and Pharmaceutical Sciences. 2012;**2012**(1):142702. DOI: 10.1155/2012/142702

[43] Ara Z, Waliullah S, Al-Otaibi ML, Alam A. A systematic review of beneficial outcomes of Omega-3 fatty acid in human musculoskeletal diseases. Endocrinology. 2022;**29**:30

Chapter 3

Osteoporosis Fracture Risk Assessment and Decision Tree Approach for Personalized Therapies

Ana Oliveira, Sara Xavier Pires, Sheila Jamal, Liliana Fonseca, Raquel Araújo, Tomás Fonseca and Ricardo Sousa

Abstract

Osteoporosis and its consequences (namely, frailty fractures) have been recognized as one of the major pandemics of the twenty-first century, due to their widespread prevalence and significant public health impact. Therapy strategies must surpass ancient rules based mainly on bone densitometry and empirical clinical features, and include updated tools on fracture risk assessment, such as novel imaging features and biomarkers, as well as clinical risk factors, such as previous fracture or history of falls. This chapter aims to guide fracture risk stratification based on the different tools available nowadays, and therapeutic approach based on the risk. We reviewed the latest evidence on fracture risk determinants and therapeutic strategies, and summarized a proposed approach to the treatment of osteoporotic patients, allowing better clinical outcomes.

Keywords: frailty fractures, fracture risk determinants, fracture risk prediction, osteoporosis treatment, individualized therapeutic approach

1. Introduction

Skeletal fragility is influenced by aging, genetics, nutrition, vitamin and mineral deficiency, lifestyle choices, smoking history, hormonal production and medication, all of which can lead to osteoporosis, a major risk for fractures [1].

Osteoporotic fractures of the hip, spine, and forearms are associated with physical deformity, chronic pain and disability, loss of independence, and, therefore, decreased quality of life [2]. Moreover, these fractures are strongly associated with low bone mineral density (BMD), are predictive of future fractures, and display an age-dependent pattern [3].

Classically, osteoporosis was determined by BMD, and more recently, the FRAX score helped to stratify fracture risk. However, many patients without densitometric osteoporosis have fragility fractures. Now we know that BMD only accounts for about 50–70% of the bone strength variation, and does not evaluate bone quality, an important determinant of bone strength [4]. New image tools, as trabecular bone score (TBS) or radiofrequency echographic multi spectrometry (REMS), biochemical biomarkers, and frailty markers, such as previous fractures or falls, add valuable information in risk stratification and help to guide the best therapeutic choice for each patient.

Selection of treatment should take into account patients and drug characteristics, regarding not only efficacy but also the celerity of the impact on bone strength.

2. Approach to the diagnosis of osteoporosis and fracture risk stratification

2.1 Bone mineral density

The diagnosis of osteoporosis by the presence of a fragility fracture is universally accepted. Dual-energy X-ray absorptiometry (DXA) was approved for the measurement of BMD by the Food and Drug Administration (FDA) in 1988 to accurately diagnose osteoporosis before a fracture occurs [3].

The World Health Organization (WHO) categorizes BMD T-scores as follows:

- Normal: −1.0 and above;
- Low bone mass (osteopenia): from −1.0 to −2.5;
- Osteoporosis: from −2.5 to −3.0;
- Severe osteoporosis: ≤ −2.5 plus fragility fracture or ≤ −3.5 without fractures [1].

With regard to risk stratifications, the lower the bone density, the higher the fracture risk.

However, BMD has a number of limitations: (i) while highly specific, BMD has low sensitivity; 60–70% of fractures occur in individuals without osteoporosis-level BMD [3]; (ii) DXA requires specialized equipment and trained personnel and may be affected by degenerative changes, previous fractures or implants [3]; (iii) cost-effectiveness of DXA screening in the general population is unclear [2]. Comorbid conditions as diabetes and chronic kidney disease, or concurrent medications as glucocorticoids, may also influence DXA results, leading to underestimation of risk [5, 6].

2.2 FRAX®

To overcome BMD limitations, risk calculators have been developed. The International Osteoporosis Foundation (IOF) and the European Society for Clinical and Economic Aspects of Osteoporosis (ESCEO) recommend expressing fracture risk as absolute 10-year probability of fracture, influenced by age, life expectancy, and risk profile [7]. FRAX® is the most widely used and validated tool (www.shef.ac.uk/FRAX) (**Figure 1**) [3].

One of the main aims for the tool was for it to be easily accessible and simple to use in primary care. FRAX® is a computer-based algorithm that estimates 10-year

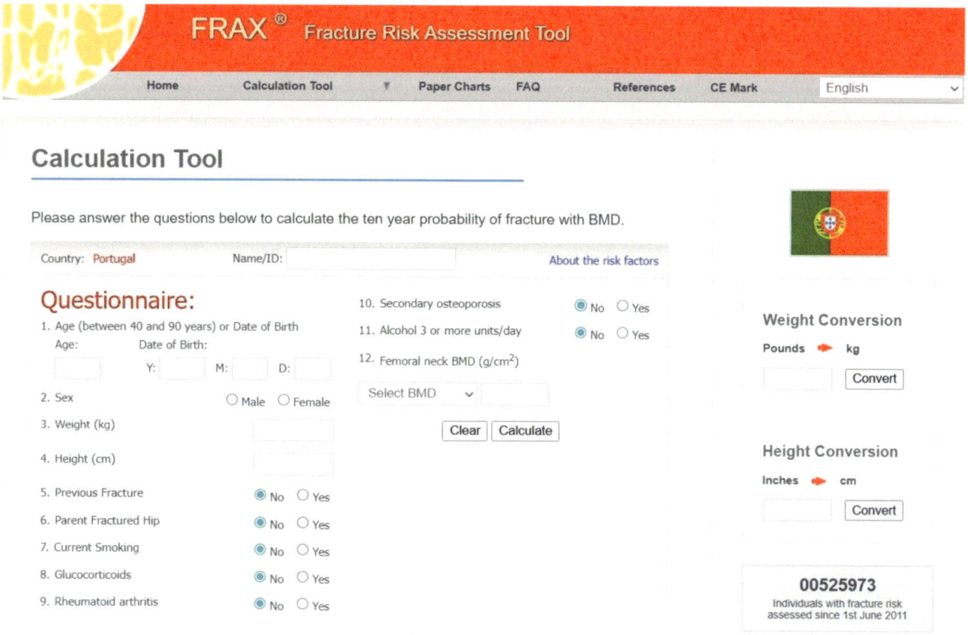

Figure 1.
FRAX, Fracture risk assessment tool, calculation tool. Available at https://frax.shef.ac.uk/FRAX/tool.aspx?country=9.

fracture probability based on clinical risk factors with or without femoral neck BMD, accommodating situations where densitometric assessment is not available [3, 8]. The ten-year time frame was selected to reflect both the typical duration of pharmacologic treatment and the temporal window during which therapeutic benefits or associated risks may manifest following treatment discontinuation [9]. It is applicable to post-menopausal women and men aged from 40 to 90 years. Its algorithm has undergone external validation in independent cohorts [10] and has been calibrated to reflect the fracture and mortality epidemiology of 67 countries, encompassing over 80% of the global population at risk [11].

However, FRAX® also has some limitations: (i) binary (yes/no) responses limit granularity (e.g., number/dose of fractures or glucocorticoids not fully captured); (ii) does not incorporate lumbar spine BMD, bone material properties, or parental fracture age [3].

2.3 FRAX plus ®

New version FRAX plus® aims to adjust probabilities for additional factors like glucocorticoid dose, lumbar spine BMD, trabecular bone score, falls history, diabetes, immigration status, and fracture recency [12]. Below are some aspects regarding concerns and pitfalls in the risk assessment.

2.3.1 Previous fractures

A history of previous fragility fractures is a well-established and independent risk factor for subsequent fractures, regardless of BMD. In the FRISBEE cohort from

Brussels, prior fragility fractures ranked as the third most important risk factor for new fractures (after age and sleeping pill intake), with a prevalence of 27%, underscoring its predictive value independent of BMD [13]. Current osteoporosis treatment guidelines recommend initiating therapy in any patient with a prior osteoporotic fracture, recognizing it as a marker of underlying bone fragility even if BMD values are not in the osteoporotic range [14].

The timing of the previous fracture critically influences risk: the imminent risk period, defined as the first two years post-fracture, carries a three- to four-fold increased fracture risk, which gradually declines by approximately 2–4% annually but remains above that of the general population [15, 16]. This imminent risk concept is now integrated into FRAX plus models to refine fracture prediction.

Fracture location also impacts risk: central fractures (vertebral, hip, proximal humerus, pelvis) confer a higher risk of subsequent fractures than peripheral fractures (forearm, ankle). Vertebral fractures notably double the risk of subsequent nonvertebral fractures and quadruple the chance of new vertebral fractures, emphasizing the importance of lateral spine imaging to detect asymptomatic vertebral fractures [17, 18].

The number of prior fractures further stratifies risk - multiple previous fractures significantly elevate the risk of future fractures, sometimes surpassing the predictive power of BMD alone [19, 20].

2.3.2 Trabecular bone score

TBS is a gray-level textural index derived from lumbar spine DXA images that reflects trabecular microarchitecture, which is often not captured by the classic methods, such as BMD [5].

Although not a direct 3D measurement, TBS correlates with parameters such as trabecular number, separation, and connectivity density. A high TBS (>1.31) indicates robust microarchitecture, while a low TBS (<1.23) reflects degraded bone quality prone to fractures [6, 21].

The ESCEO has endorsed TBS as a complementary tool to BMD and clinical risk factors, improving fracture risk prediction in primary and secondary osteoporosis, helping clinical decisions. Current data support the role of the TBS in the assessment of fragility fracture risk in patients with a variety of secondary causes of osteoporosis independently of BMD, in particular chronic kidney disease, parathyroid disease, and rheumatic diseases with chronic inflammation. It also adds predictive value beyond lumbar spine BMD, particularly useful in conditions where BMD underestimates risk [5, 6]. Importantly, TBS is less affected by osteoarthritis than BMD, increasing its reliability [22].

However, this is a score that may be interfered by age (little changes are observed between 30 and 45 years old, with progressive decrease in advancing age) and soft tissue thickness (but the improvement and reliability of the algorithm has turned this less relevant) [5, 21].

Therapeutically, anabolic agents such as parathyroid hormone analogues and romosozumab have demonstrated significant TBS improvements, whereas antiresorptives like bisphosphonates and selective estrogen receptor modulators (SERMs) primarily stabilize microarchitecture with minimal TBS change [22]. Thus, TBS assists in stratifying treatment, guiding anabolic-first strategies in very high-risk patients. Recent studies also explore TBS applicability beyond the lumbar spine to other sites like the hip and distal femur [6].

2.3.3 Glucocorticoid therapy

High-dose or long-term glucocorticoid use is the most common cause of secondary osteoporosis, impairing both bone quantity and quality and leading to fractures at higher BMD values than in non-users. Bone loss begins early (within 3–6 months) and is dose-dependent [23–25]. Daily doses >15–30 mg or cumulative doses >5 g/year of prednisolone significantly increase fracture risk. FRAX underestimates fracture risk in glucocorticoid users, as it only accounts for ≥5 mg/day use for 3+ months. Greater adjustments are needed for higher doses (>7.5 mg/day) [24, 26, 27]. Some international guidelines recommend osteoporosis treatment for all patients on ≥2.5 mg/day of prednisolone for more than 3 months, with treatment choice based on individual risk level [25, 27]. Bone loss partially reverses after glucocorticoid withdrawal, but may not return to baseline levels [24].

2.3.4 Type 2 diabetes mellitus

Type 2 diabetes increases fracture risk (both vertebral and nonvertebral) despite normal or elevated BMD, a phenomenon known as the "diabetic paradox." Diabetic bone shows increased cortical porosity and compromised bone microstructure, especially in trabecular bone, leading to reduced bone strength. Imaging studies reveal preserved trabecular structure but impaired cortical integrity, influenced by changes in weight-bearing patterns, turning tools, such as TBS, which are better in risk assessment for those patients [28–30]. Diabetics exhibit low bone turnover, with suppressed bone turnover markers, likely due to insulin resistance. Bone biopsies confirm this low turnover state [30]. Other contributing factors include longer disease duration, poor physical function, and increased fall risk, especially in older adults [28, 29]. In high-risk patients, hypoglycemia-inducing medications should be avoided due to their link with falls and fracture risk [29, 30].

2.3.5 Fall history and prevention

Falling is a major health problem in old age. Every year, 30% of the elderly fall once, and 15% at least twice. From this, 5–10% result in a fracture. Indeed, up to 90% of all fractures result from a fall. Besides fractures, other major injuries, physical disability, functional impairment, dependency in activities of daily living, institutionalization, increased morbidity, and mortality are significant results from falls [31, 32]. The costs associated with all those problems are significant to the health care systems [31].

The most important predictor for falling is having a history of falling. The probability of a fracture as a consequence of the fall is directly related to cone strength. As such, assessment of fracture risk is indicated in all patients with high fall risk and with a previous history of falls. Patients with high risk for fractures should be evaluated for the risk of falls, and preventive strategies should be undertaken [31]. Other risk factors for falls include female sex, sarcopenia, fear of falling, impaired cognition, mobility, and gait [32].

Systematic assessment of fall risk in older adults is essential. From the age of 65, all patients should undergo opportunistic assessments in a primary care setting to evaluate fall risk, based on fall history, fear of falling, and signs of unsteadiness [33]. After identifying fall risk, strategies to prevent falls are crucial. A combination of non-pharmacological strategies, including lifestyle modification and exercise, can significantly reduce fall and fracture risks (**Table 1**) [33–36].

General approach	• Non-pharmacological strategies, like promoting adequate intake of vitamin D and protein, support bone strength and reduce fracture risk
Low risk No recent falls or concerns about balance	• Health promotion (exercise, nutrition, lifestyle) • Physical activity goals: o 150–300 minutes/week moderate-intensity OR o 75–150 minutes/week vigorous-intensity • Regular vision and hearing checks
Intermediate risk Gait speed ≤0.8 m/s OR one fall in the past year	• Individualized exercise programs focused on: o Balance, strength, functional movements (e.g., sit-to-stand, stepping, multidirectional walking) o Use of resistance (e.g., weights) to promote neuromuscular adaptation • Regular review and progression of exercise intensity.
High risk More than one fall in the past year, presence of frailty, or injury from a fall	• Requires a comprehensive multifactorial assessment including: o Medical history and fall circumstances o Cardiovascular and neurological exams o Vision, hearing, gait, and balance testing o Medication review and deprescribing (e.g., benzodiazepines) o Screening for pain, incontinence, depression, cognitive decline, substance use, and nutrition o Evaluation of the home environment for hazards • Multidisciplinary, tailored to individual needs and preferences • Exercise recommendations: o At least three times/week for 12 weeks o Gradual progression to maintenance phase with independent practice o Level of supervision depends on frailty o Address cardiovascular, vestibular, and visual issues. • Provide assistive walking devices if needed. • Conduct home safety assessments with follow-up and support for hazard reduction.

Table 1.
Fall risk stratification and specific interventions.

2.3.6 Lumbar spine bone mineral density

FRAX plus® also considers the T-score from the lumbar spine, making a better prediction of fracture risk in those patients with lumbar spine osteoporosis and normal or low decrease (osteopenia) BMD of the femur.

2.3.7 Hip axis length

Hip axis length (HAL) is defined as the distance from the base of the greater trochanter to the inner pelvic brim. HAL independently predicts hip fracture risk, particularly in younger, non-osteoporotic women, supplementing BMD and FRAX assessments [37].

2.4 New diagnostic and fracture risk assessment tools

2.4.1 Radiofrequency echographic multi spectrometry

REMS is a novel, portable, radiation-free ultrasound technology validated for assessing bone health at the lumbar spine and proximal femur. The clinician places the ultrasound probe at the hip and lumbar spine, adjusts the depth and the focus of the transducer, and the software detects bone interfaces and the regions of interest for bone evaluation. The REMS algorithm adjusts the results to gender, age, site, and body mass index. It generates BMD-equivalent T- and Z-scores and introduces a fragility score (FS) quantifying bone quality from 0 (normal) to 100 (maximum fragility), predictive of fracture risk over five years [38–40].

REMS addresses limitations of DXA by minimizing artifacts from spinal degeneration, vertebral fractures, metal implants, and aortic calcifications, which may artificially elevate DXA BMD. Studies suggest REMS performs comparably or superiorly to DXA for osteoporosis diagnosis and fracture risk prediction, with special advantages in populations with altered bone metabolism and where DXA underestimates risk [38–40].

Its portability facilitates bedside assessment of frail or post-fracture patients and enables radiation-free, frequent monitoring in populations like children, pregnant women, and those on medications affecting bone. REMS may improve adherence monitoring by providing timely feedback on treatment response. Its high precision allows short-term monitoring, being capable of detecting bone mass changes in at-risk populations, such as in patients treated with aromatase inhibitors or corticosteroids, or in pregnancy-associated osteoporosis. While promising, further longitudinal studies are needed to fully define its clinical role [39, 40].

2.4.2 Bone turnover markers

Bone turnover markers (BTMs) reflect the dynamic balance of bone resorption and formation, with resorption markers such as C-terminal telopeptide of type I collagen (CTX-I) and formation markers like procollagen type 1 amino-terminal propeptide (PINP) being most studied [41–44]. Elevated BTMs have been associated with increased fracture risk in some studies, yet evidence remains inconsistent due to methodological variability and confounding factors (age, circadian rhythm, comorbidities) [41, 42].

BTMs have limited utility in routine fracture risk prediction, especially in elderly patients and those with type 2 diabetes, who typically exhibit a low bone turnover state. However, BTMs are valuable in monitoring osteoporosis treatment adherence and efficacy, as they respond rapidly to therapeutic changes [41–44].

2.4.3 Quantitative computed tomography

Quantitative Computed Tomography (QCT) offers 3D volumetric assessment of bone geometry and density, providing insights into cortical and trabecular compartments separately, with growing use in specialized settings. Accessibility, costs, and exposure to radiation may limit its use.

3. Management of patients at low, high, and very high risk of osteoporotic fractures

As previously detailed, fracture risk can be calculated with FRAX® and stratified into three categories: low, high, and very high. According to the zone category (**Figure 2**), different strategies should be implemented:

- Red zone: indicates very high risk; treatment with an initial course of anabolic therapy followed by antiresorptive agents is recommended.
- Green zone: indicates low risk; management includes lifestyle advice, adequate calcium and vitamin D intake, and consideration of menopausal hormone therapy (MHT).
- Orange zone: Represents intermediate risk; further assessment with femoral neck BMD is required, followed by recalculation of FRAX probability:
  - o Reclassification to the red zone indicates a very high risk.
  - o Persistence in the orange zone suggests high risk, for which antiresorptive therapy is appropriate.
  - o Reclassification to the green zone confirms low risk, including patients who were initially borderline.

Individuals with a prior fragility fracture are automatically considered at least high risk and potentially very high risk, depending on FRAX probability [46].

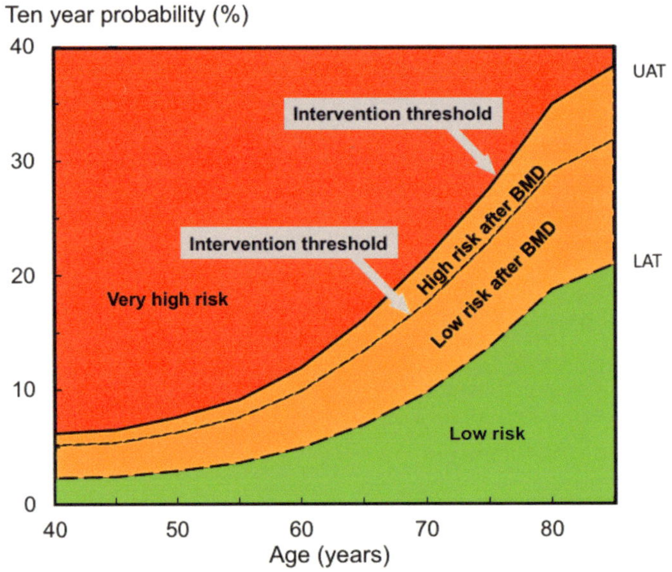

Figure 2.
Infographic representation of fracture risk stratification in postmenopausal women based on FRAX®-derived 10-year probability of major osteoporotic fracture, using clinical risk factors (CRFs) alone at the initial assessment. Adapted from [45].

The criteria defining high and very high fracture risk are summarized in **Table 2** [46–50].

All individuals, regardless of risk category, should receive education on lifestyle modifications, including adequate calcium and vitamin D intake. In low-risk patients, menopausal hormone therapy (MHT) and SERMs may be considered. For individuals categorized as high or very high risk, the American Association of Clinical Endocrinology (AACE) strongly recommends the initiation of pharmacologic therapy.

The diagrams below (**Figures 3** and **4**) systematically summarize the treatment of high- and very-high-risk patients.

High risk	• T-scores between −1.0 and – 2.5 and a history of fragility fracture of the hip or spine • T-scores between −1.0 and – 2.5 and a FRAX® 10-year probability of major osteoporotic fracture ≥20% or 10-year probability of hip fracture ≥3% in the U.S • In some countries (such as Portugal), lower thresholds are applied - FRAX® 10-year probability of ≥9% for major osteoporotic fractures or ≥ 2.5% for hip fractures. In other countries or regions, treatment decisions should be guided by the corresponding country-specific intervention thresholds, which reflect local epidemiology and cost-effectiveness considerations
Very high risk	• Recent fracture (e.g., within the past 12 months) • Those who have fractures while on approved osteoporosis therapy • Multiple fractures • Fractures while on drugs, causing skeletal harm (e.g., long-term glucocorticoids) • Those with a very low T-score (e.g., less than −3.0) • High risk of falls or history of injurious falls • Those with a very high fracture probability by FRAX® (e.g., major osteoporosis fracture >30%, hip fracture >4.5%) or other validated fracture risk algorithms

Table 2.
Definition of high and very high risk.

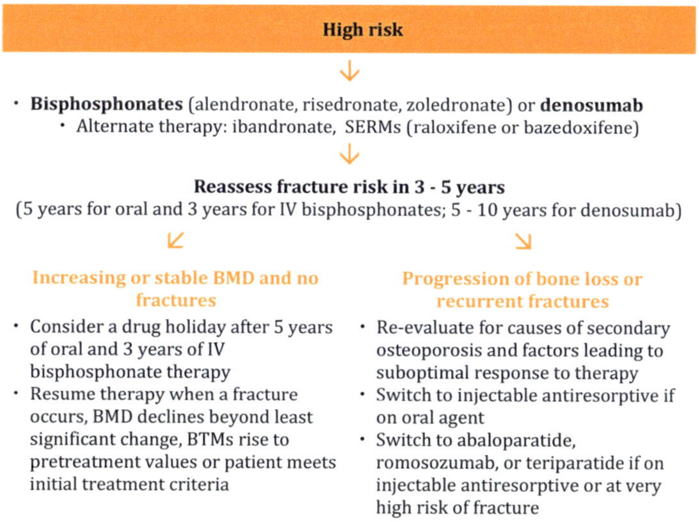

Figure 3.
Treatment of high-risk patients.

Very high risk

Consider anabolic agent followed by inhibitor of bone resorption

Romosozumab for 1 year

Abaloparatide or **teriparatide** for up to 2 years

Sequential therapy with oral or injectable antiresorptive agent

If anabolic agents are not available, consider:

- Denosumab
- Zoledronate (If stable, continue therapy for 6 years. Consider a drug holiday after 6 years of IV zoledronate or switch to denosumab according to reassessment of fracture risk. If drug holiday, a weaker antiresorptive such as raloxifene could be used)

Figure 4.
Treatment of very high-risk patients.

			Reduction of fracture risk		
			Vertebral	**Nonvertebral**	**Hip**
Antiresorptive therapy	Bisphospho-nates	Alendronate	Yes	Yes	Yes
		Risedronate	Yes	Yes	Yes
		Ibandronate	Yes	NED[a]	NED[a]
		Zoledronate	Yes	Yes	Yes
	RANK-ligand inhibitor (monoclonal antibody)	Denosumab	Yes	Yes	Yes
	SERMs	Raloxifene	Yes	NED[a]	NED[a]
		Bazedoxifene	Yes	NED[a]	NED[a]
Anabolic agents	Parathyroid Hormone Analogues	Teriparatide	Yes	Yes	NED[a]
		Abaloparatide	Yes	Yes	NED[a]
	Sclerostin inhibitor (monoclonal antibody)	Romosozumab	Yes	[b]	[b]

[a] *The lack of demonstrable effect at these sites should be considered in the context that the studies may not have been adequately powered.*
[b] *Romosozumab significantly enhanced BMD gains over alendronate after the initial 12 months. Furthermore, romosozumab showed superiority in reducing the risks of nonvertebral and hip fractures by 48%, 27%, 19%, and 38%, respectively. Real-World Evidence from Japan that had nonvertebral and hip fractures as the primary outcome. No significant difference between romosozumab and teriparatide in preventing nonvertebral or hip fractures was found [51].*

Table 3.
Summary of evidence for reduction of risk with pharmacologic agents. NED—no effect demonstrated.

	Dose	Adverse effects	Contraindications
Antiresorptive therapy			
Alendronate	Oral: 70 mg weekly or 10 mg daily	• Esophageal or GI intolerance • MSK discomfort • Rare: AFF, ONJ	• CrCl <30–35 mL/min • Esophageal abnormalities • Inability to be upright >30 min • Hypocalcemia
Risedronate	Oral: 35 mg weekly or 150 mg monthly or 5 mg daily		
Ibandronate	Oral: 2.5 mg daily or 150 mg monthly Intravenous: 3 mg IV every 3 months		
Zoledronate	Intravenous: 5 mg yearly	• Transient flu-like symptoms • Hypocalcemia • Renal toxicity • Rare: AFF, ONJ	• CrCl <35 mL/min • Hypocalcemia
Denosumab	Subcutaneous: 60 mg every 6 months	• Hypocalcemia • Dermatitis, infections • MSK discomfort • Rare: AFF, ONJ	• Hypocalcemia
Hormonal therapy			
Menopausal hormonal therapy	Multiple regimens	• VTE, CVD, stroke • Breast cancer	• VTE, CVD, stroke, estrogen-dependent tumors, abnormal vaginal bleeding, active liver disease
Raloxifene (SERM)	Oral: 60 mg daily	• VTE, CVD, stroke • Vasomotor symptoms, leg cramps	• VTE, CVD, stroke, abnormal vaginal bleeding
Bazedoxifene (SERM)	Oral: 20 mg daily	• VTE, CVD, stroke • Vasomotor symptoms, leg cramps	• VTE, CVD, stroke, abnormal vaginal bleeding
Anabolic agents			
Teriparatide	Subcutaneous: 20 μg daily for 24 months	• Orthostatic hypotension, nausea • Hypercalcemia, hypercalciuria • MSK discomfort	• CrCl <30 mL/min • Bone malignancy, Paget disease, previous skeletal radiation • Hypercalcemia disorder • Unexplained elevated ALP
Abalopara-tide	Subcutaneous: 80 μg daily	• Orthostatic hypotension, nausea • Hypercalcemia, hypercalciuria • Dizziness, headache, palpitations, fatigue, upper abdominal pain	• CrCl <30 mL/min • Bone malignancy, Paget disease, previous skeletal radiation • Hypercalcemia disorder • Unexplained elevated ALP

	Dose	Adverse effects	Contraindications
Romosozu-mab	Subcutaneous: 210 mg monthly for 12 months	• Myocardial infarction, stroke • Hypocalcemia • MSK discomfort • Rare: AFF, ONJ	• Previous myocardial infarction or stroke • Hypocalcemia

AFF—atypical femoral fracture, ALP—alkaline phosphatase, CrCl—creatinine clearance, CVD—cardiovascular disease, GI—gastrointestinal, IV—intravenous, MSK—musculoskeletal, ONJ—osteonecrosis of the jaw, RANK—receptor activator of nuclear factor κ-β, VTE—venous thromboembolism.

Table 4.
Medications for the treatment of osteoporosis.

Tables 3 and **4** provide a comprehensive summary of the pharmacological agents currently approved for the treatment of osteoporosis. These tables categorize the available therapies by drug class—such as antiresorptives and anabolic agents—and present key clinical information, including the level of evidence supporting fracture risk reduction across different skeletal sites (e.g., vertebral, nonvertebral, and hip fractures). Additionally, they outline standard dosing regimens, routes of administration (oral, subcutaneous, or intravenous), and relevant contraindications that may influence treatment selection [46–49, 51, 52]. This structured overview is intended to support clinical decision-making by enabling personalized, evidence-based therapeutic choices tailored to the patient's risk profile and clinical context.

These tables categorize the available therapies by drug class—such as antiresorptives and anabolic agents—and present key clinical information, including the level of evidence supporting fracture risk reduction across different skeletal sites (e.g., vertebral, nonvertebral, and hip fractures). Additionally, they outline standard dosing regimens, routes of administration (oral, subcutaneous, or intravenous), and relevant contraindications that may influence treatment selection [46–49, 51, 52]. This structured overview is intended to support clinical decision-making by enabling personalized, evidence-based therapeutic choices tailored to the patient's risk profile and clinical context.

4. Conclusion

Classical stratification of fracture risk using FRAX® is still the gold standard for fracture risk assessment, enabling sequential and tailored osteoporosis management:

- Low-risk patients receive lifestyle advice and possibly MHT.
- High-risk patients benefit from antiresorptive agents.
- Very high-risk patients require anabolic therapy followed by antiresorptive maintenance.

However, nowadays a number of other clinical, analytical, and imaging features are also known to be important determinants of fracture risk, and should be taken into account, allowing a better decision on treatment choice, with improvements in patient outcomes, and reduced burden of fragility fractures globally.

Acknowledgements

Ricardo Rodrigues Pinto, Orthopedics and Traumatology Department, Unidade Local de Saúde de Santo António, and Instituto de Ciências Biomédicas Abel Salazar (ICBAS), Universidade do Porto, Porto, Portugal.

Author details

Ana Oliveira[1*], Sara Xavier Pires[1], Sheila Jamal[1], Liliana Fonseca[2,8], Raquel Araújo[3], Tomás Fonseca[4,8,9] and Ricardo Sousa[5,6,7,8,9]

1 Internal Medicine Department, Unidade Local de Saúde de Santo António, Porto, Portugal

2 Endocrinology Department, Unidade Local de Saúde de Santo António, Porto, Portugal

3 Physical Medicine and Rehabilitation Department, Unidade Local de Saúde de Santo António, Porto, Portugal

4 Clinical Immunology Unit, Unidade Local de Saúde de Santo António, Porto, Portugal

5 Orthopedics and Traumatology Department, Unidade Local de Saúde de Santo António, Porto, Portugal

6 Porto Bone and Joint Infection Group (GRIP), Unidade Local de Saúde de Santo António, Porto, Portugal

7 Orthopedics and Department, Hospital Lusíadas, Porto, Portugal

8 Instituto de Ciências Biomédicas Abel Salazar (ICBAS), Universidade do Porto, Porto, Portugal

9 Unit for Multidisciplinary Research in Biomedicine (UMIB), Instituto de Ciências Biomédicas Abel Salazar (ICBAS), Universidade do Porto, Porto, Portugal

*Address all correspondence to: oliveira.anamp@gmail.com

References

[1] Yedavally-Yellayi S, Ho AM, Patalinghug EM. Update on osteoporosis. Primary Care: Clinic in Office Practice. 2019;**46**(1):175-190

[2] Yong E-L, Logan S. Menopausal osteoporosis: Screening, prevention and treatment. Singapore Medical Journal. 2021;**62**(4):159-166

[3] Schini M, Johansson H, Harvey NC, Lorentzon M, Kanis JA, McCloskey EV. An overview of the use of the fracture risk assessment tool (FRAX) in osteoporosis. Journal of Endocrinological Investigation. 2023;**47**(3):501-511

[4] Diez-Perez A, Brandi ML, Al-Daghri N, et al. Radiofrequency echographic multi-spectrometry for the in-vivo assessment of bone strength: State of the art—outcomes of an expert consensus meeting organized by the ESCEO. Aging Clinical and Experimental Research. 2019;**31**:1375-1389

[5] Harvey NC, Gluer CC, Binkley N, et al. Trabecular bone score (TBS) as a new complementary approach for osteoporosis evaluation in clinical practice. Bone. 2015;**78**:216-224

[6] Shevroja E, Reginster J-Y, Lamy O, et al. Update on the clinical use of TBS in the management of osteoporosis: Results of an expert group meeting organized by the ESCEO, and the IOF under the auspices of WHO collaborating Center for Epidemiology of musculoskeletal health and aging. Osteoporosis International. 2023;**34**:1501-1529

[7] Kanis JA, Cooper C, Rizzoli R, Reginster J-Y. European guidance for the diagnosis and management of osteoporosis in postmenopausal women. Osteoporosis International. 2018;**30**(1):3-44

[8] Siris SA, Ethel S. Primary care use of FRAX: Absolute fracture risk assessment in postmenopausal women and older men. Postgraduate Medicine. 2010;**122**(1):82-90

[9] Kanis J. World Health Organization scientific group 2007. Assessment of osteoporosis at the primary health care level. In: Technical Report, World Health Organization Collaborating Centre for Metabolic Bone Diseases. Sheffield, UK: University of Sheffield; 2007

[10] Kanis JA, Oden A, Johnell O, et al. The use of clinical risk factors enhances the performance of BMD in the prediction of hip and osteoporotic fractures in men and women. Osteoporosis International. 2007;**18**(8):1033-1046

[11] Kanis JA, Harvey NC, Cooper C, Johansson H, Odén A, McCloskey EV. A systematic review of intervention thresholds based on FRAX: A report prepared for the national osteoporosis guideline group and the international osteoporosis foundation. Archives of Osteoporosis. 2016;**11**(1):1-48

[12] McCloskey EV, Harvey NC, Johansson H, Lorentzon M, Liu E, Vandenput L, et al. Fracture risk assessment by the FRAX model. Climacteric. 2022;**25**(1):22-28

[13] Capelle SI, Ramon I, Dekelver C, et al. Distribution of clinical risk factors for fracture in a Brussels cohort of postmenopausal women: The FRISBEE study and comparison with other major cohort studies. Maturitas. 2017;**106**:1-7

[14] Kanis JA, Johansson H, McCloskey EV, et al. Previous fracture and subsequent fracture risk: A

meta-analysis to update FRAX. Osteoporosis International. 2023;**34**(12):2027-2045

[15] McCloskey EV, Borgstrom F, Cooper C, Harvey NC, Javaid MK, Lorentzon M, et al. Short time horizons for fracture prediction tools: Time for a rethink. Osteoporosis International. 2021;**32**(6):1019-1025

[16] Iconaru L, Charles A, Beleanu F, et al. Prediction of an imminent fracture after an index fracture—Models derived from the Frisbee cohort. Journal of Bone and Mineral Research. 2021;**37**(1):59-67

[17] Iconaru L, Moreau M, Baleanu F, et al. Risk factors for imminent fractures: A substudy of the FRISBEE cohort. Osteoporosis International. 2021;**32**(6):1093-1101

[18] Johansson L, Johansson H, Axelsson KF, et al. Improved fracture risk prediction by adding VFA-identified vertebral fracture data to BMD by DXA and clinical risk factors used in FRAX. Osteoporosis International. 2022;**33**(8):1725-1738

[19] Lunt M, O'Neill TW, Felsenberg D, et al. Characteristics of a prevalent vertebral deformity predict subsequent vertebral fracture: Results from the European prospective osteoporosis study (EPOS). Bone. 2003;**33**(4):505-513

[20] Delmas PD, Genant HK, Crans GG, et al. Severity of prevalent vertebral fractures and the risk of subsequent vertebral and nonvertebral fractures: Results from the MORE trial. Bone. 2003;**33**(4):522-532

[21] Rajan R, Cherian KE, Kappor N, Paul TV. Trabecular bone score—An emerging tool in the management of osteoporosis. Indian Journal of Endocrinology and Metabolism. 2020;**24**:237-243

[22] Miedany YE, Elwakil W, Abu-Zaid MH, Mahran S. Update on the utility of trabecular bone score (TBS) in clinical practice for the management of osteoporosis: A systematic review by the Egyptian academy of bone and muscle health. Egyptian Rheumatology and Rehabilitation. 2024;**51**:18

[23] Chen M, Fu W, Xu H, Liu C-J. Pathogenic mechanisms of glucocorticoid-induced osteoporosis. Cytokine & Growth Factor Reviews. 2023;**70**:54-66

[24] Compston J. Glucocorticoid-induced osteoporosis: An update. Endocrine. 2018;**61**(1):7-16

[25] Tanaka Y, Soen S, Hirata S, et al. The 2023 guidelines for the management and treatment of glucocorticoid-induced osteoporosis. Journal of Bone and Mineral Metabolism. 2024;**42**(2):143-154

[26] De Vries F, Bracke M, Leufkens H, Lammers J-WJ, Cooper C, Staa TV. Fracture risk with intermittent high-dose oral glucocorticoid therapy. Arthritis & Rheumatism. 2007;**56**(1):208-214

[27] Humphrey MB, Russell L, Danila MI, et al. 2022 American college of rheumatology guideline for the prevention and treatment of glucocorticoid-induced osteoporosi. Arthritis and Rheumatology. 2023;**75**(12):2088-2012

[28] Zoulakis M, Johansson L, Litsne H, et al. Type 2 diabetes and fracture risk in older women. Diabetes and Endocrinology. 2024;**7**(8):e2425106

[29] Martiniakova M, Biro R, Penzes N, et al. Links among obesity, type 2 diabetes mellitus, and osteoporosis: Bone as a target. International Journal of Molecular Sciences. 2024;**25**(9):4827

[30] Sheu A, Greenfield JR, White CP, Center JR. Assessment and treatment of osteoporosis and fractures in type 2 diabetes. Trends in Endocrinology and Metabolism. 2022;**33**(5):333-344

[31] Peeters G, van Schoor NM, Lips P. Fall risk: The clinical relevance of falls and how to integrate fall risk with fracture risk. Best Practice & Research Clinical Rheumatology. 2009;**23**(6):794-804

[32] Yeung S, Reijnierse E, Pham V, et al. Sarcopenia and its association with falls and fractures in older adults: A systematic review and meta-analysis. Journal of Cachexia, Sarcopenia and Muscle. 2019;**10**:485-500

[33] Montero-Odasso M, van der Velde N, Martin F, et al. World guidelines for falls prevention and management for older adults: A global initiative. Age and Ageing. 2022;**51**:1-36

[34] Hopewll S, Adedire O, Copsey GJ, et al. Multifactorial and multiple component interventions for preventing falls in older people living in the community (review). Cochrane Database of Systematic Reviews. 2018;**7**:CD012221

[35] Gillespie LD, Robertson MC, Gillespie WJ, et al. Interventions for preventing falls in older people living in the community (review). Cochrane Database of Systematic Reviews. 2012;**9**:CD007146

[36] McClure RJ, Turner C, Peel N, Spinks A, Eakin E, Hughes K. Population-based interventions for the prevention of fall-related injuries in older people (review). Cochrane Database of Systematic Reviews. 2005;**1**:CD004441

[37] Leslie WD, Lix LM, Morin SN, et al. Hip axis length is a FRAX- and bone density-independent risk factor for hip fracture in women. The Journal of Clinical Endocrinology & Metabolism. 2015;**100**(5):2063-2070

[38] Al Refaie A, Baldassini L, Mondillo C, et al. Radiofrequency echographic multi spectrometry (R.E.M.S.): New frontiers for ultrasound use in the assessment of bone status-a current picture. Diagnostics. 2023;**13**(10):1666

[39] Icatoiu E, Vladulescu-Trandafir A-I, Groşeanu L-M, et al. Radiofrequency echographic multi spectrometry—A novel tool in the diagnosis of osteoporosis and prediction of fragility fractures: A systematic review. Diagnostics. 2025;**15**(5):555

[40] Fuggle NR, Reginster J-Y, Al-Daghri N, et al. Radiofrequency echographic multi spectrometry (REMS) in the diagnosis and management of osteoporosis: State of the art. Aging Clinical and Experimental Research. 2024;**36**(1):135

[41] Di Medio L, Brandi ML. Advances in bone turnover markers. Advances in Clinical Chemistry. 2021;**105**:101-140

[42] Ivaska KK, McGuigan FE, Malmgren L, et al. Bone turnover marker profiling and fracture risk in older women: Fracture risk from age 75 to 90. Calcified Tissue International. 2022;**111**:288-299

[43] Massera D, Xu S, Walker MD, et al. Biochemical markers of bone turnover and risk of incident hip fracture in older women: The cardiovascular health study. Osteoporosis International. 2019;**30**(9):1755-1765

[44] Morris HA, Eastell R, Jorgensen NR, et al. Clinical usefulness of bone turnover marker concentrations in osteoporosis. Clinica Chimica Acta. 2017;**467**:34-41

[45] Kanis JA et al. Algorithm for the management of patients at low, high and very high risk of osteoporotic fractures. Osteoporosis International. 2020;**31**:1-12. DOI: 10.1007/s00198-019-05176-3

[46] Kanis JA, Harvey NC, McCloskey E, et al. Algorithm for the management of patients at low, high and very high risk of osteoporotic fractures. Osteoporosis International. 2019;**31**(1):1-12

[47] Camacho PM, Petak SM, Binkley N, et al. American association of clinical endocrinologists/American college of endocrinology clinical practice guidelines for the diagnosis and treatment of postmenopausal osteoporosis—2020 update. Endocrine Practice. 2020;**26**(1):1-46

[48] Morin SN, Feldman S, Funnell L, et al. Clinical practice guideline for management of osteoporosis and fracture prevention in Canada: 2023 update. Canadian Medical Association Journal. 2023;**195**(39):E1333-E1348

[49] Shoback D, Rosen CJ, Black DM, Cheung AM, Murad MH, Eastell R. Pharmacological management of osteoporosis in postmenopausal women: An endocrine society guideline update. The Journal of Clinical Endocrinology & Metabolism. 2020;**105**(3):dgaa048

[50] Marques A, Rodrigues AM, Romeu JC, et al. Recomendações multidisciplinares portuguesas sobre o pedido de DXA e indicação de tratamento de prevenção das fraturas de fragilidade. Revista Portuguesa de Medicina Geral e Familiar. 2016;**32**(6):425-441

[51] Masuda S, Fukasawa T, Matsuda S, Yoshida S, Kawakami K. Comparative effectiveness and cardiovascular safety of romosozumab versus teriparatide in patients with osteoporosis: A population-based cohort study. Osteoporosis International. 2024;**35**(12):2165-2174

[52] G-Saag K, Petersen J, Brandi ML, et al. Romosozumab or alendronate for fracture prevention in women with osteoporosis. New England Journal of Medicine. 2017;**377**(15):1417-1427

Chapter 4

Nutrition in Osteoporosis: Prevention and Management

Samiya Khan, Bhagyashree Parab and Sadaf Hasan

Abstract

Osteoporosis is a common public health issue, prevalent in one in four women and one in eight men over the age of 50. Decreased bones mass and micro-architecture are the main characteristics of osteoporosis, which make bones more fragile leading to the risk of fractures. Frailty to fracture is linked to morbidity, mortality, and disability, which has become an important global health issue. Recent data have shown that optimum nutrition which include protein, dietary fiber, essential fatty acids, minerals (calcium, phosphorus, magnesium), vitamins (vitamin D, C, K), and physical activity, plays a key role in achieving the maximum bone mineral density (BMD), supports bone health, and reduces fracture risk. The effects of these macro- and micronutrients take place at various aspects of bone metabolism, mineralization, and muscle function, which impact on bone strength. Thus, keeping up a healthy lifestyle, including sufficient nutrition and exercise, can significantly improve the overall bone health and decrease the risk of osteoporosis.

Keywords: bone mineral density, osteoporosis, nutrition, physical activity, lifestyle

1. Introduction

Osteoporosis is a commonly prevalent metabolic bone disorder characterized by a reduced bone mass and density, accompanied by declined bone matrix and mineralization, leading to decreased bone mass and an increased risk of fractures [1]. The World Health Organization (WHO) defines osteoporosis as a "progressive systemic skeletal disorder characterized by low bone mass and deterioration of the microarchitecture of bone tissue, leading to increased fragility and susceptibility to fractures" [2]. From the past few years, this condition had been described as a syndrome accompanied by osteopenia, vertebral fractures, and back pain. Nevertheless, osteoporosis is now recognized as a skeletal disorder associated with significant metabolic changes in both bone and overall body homeostasis [3]. It is more prevalent in women and geriatric population, but sometime it is also seen in young adults [4]. Osteoporosis is classified into two categories: primary, which includes idiopathic, senile, or postmenopausal osteoporosis, and secondary, which occurs in both men and women as a result of a specific primary condition, such as Cushing's syndrome [1].

Osteoporosis affects approximately 200 million individuals globally [5], and it is increasingly common among the aging population, which is a gradual and chronic bone disorder. The occurrence of osteoporosis is significantly higher in people with aged 60 and older (37.0%) compared to those younger than 60 (12.5%). The prevalence can differ by region and country, and in certain areas, the higher rates of osteoporosis are seen than others. For example, a study found the highest prevalence in Africa [6]. While it can impact population of any age or ethnicity, women after menopause face a higher risk due to reduced estrogen levels [7]. This condition affects 10% of the global population and 30% of women who have gone through menopause [8]. In comparison with adults, children and teenagers experience lower rates of secondary osteoporosis, which is an emerging concern. Secondary osteoporosis, often linked to chronic medical conditions or prolonged medication use, occurs more frequently than primary osteoporosis. Some studies suggest that the incidence of osteopenia and osteoporosis among specific age groups varies between 12 and 40% [9]. As a result, the World Health Organization characterizes osteoporosis as a "global health issue" and refers to it as the silent epidemic of the twenty-first century because of its effects on public health [10].

2. Normal bone homeostasis

Over the years, research has demonstrated the crucial role of bone as an organ that constantly interacts with and controls several other tissues. In addition to its traditional functions in movement, internal organ protection, and mineral homeostasis, bone also helps control glucose metabolism and energy expenditure, affects male fertility, and affects cognitive abilities by secreting osteocalcin by osteoblasts. To perform its functions, bone undergoes continuous cycles of modeling and remodeling [11]. During modeling and growth period, bone changes its shape and size for mechanical adaptation, independent bone formation, and resorption at separate sites, where during remodeling bone resorption and formation occur at the same site, which is a crucial process for repairing damage, maintaining structural integrity, and regulating calcium and phosphate balance. Bone remodeling plays a crucial role in bone homeostasis; deranged remodeling increases bone resorption over bone formation, which is a mechanism leading to bone disorders, such as osteoporosis. The main bone cells that are involved in bone modeling and remodeling are of three types: osteoclasts (bone resorbing), osteoblasts (bone forming), and osteocytes, former osteoblasts embedded in bone, now recognized as the key regulators of bone homeostasis.

To maintain the bone mass, remodeling relies on a balance between the amount of bone resorbed by osteoclasts and the amount of bone formed by osteoblasts. Receptor activator of nuclear factor-kB (RANK) and its ligand RANKL maintain the regulation of bone cells, while its decoy receptor osteoprotegerin (OPG) is primarily involved in regulating osteoclast differentiation, activation, and survival, and bone remodeling depends on this mechanism [12]. Bone morphogenetic proteins (BMP) and wingless-related integration site (Wnt) signaling pathway proteins regulate osteoblasts and their differentiation. They initiate the canonical Wnt signaling pathway by binding to the transmembrane proteins frizzled receptor (Fzd) and LDL receptor-related protein (LRP) 5 or 6 [13].

Osteocytes are the most abundant bone cells, which are vital for maintaining the equilibrium of minerals in the bones. These cells regulate calcium and phosphate levels and play an important part in bone remodeling by coordinating with osteoblasts and osteoclasts through a complex network. This network connects osteocytes to the bone vasculature, allowing them to influence bone cell activity through effector proteins, such as sclerostin (which inhibits Wnt signaling) and RANKL (which promotes osteoclast formation). In certain conditions, like immobilization, hyperparathyroidism, and lactation, osteocytes can remodel their immediate environment by resorbing or depositing bone [14]. Therefore, an imbalance between any of the bone cells, such as osteoblast, osteoclast, and osteocytes, can lead to osteoporosis, causing weakened bone and increasing the chances of fracture [15].

3. Pathophysiology of osteoporosis

Earlier studies typically emphasized endocrine factors, such as vitamin D deficiency, reduced food consumption, estrogen deficit, and secondary hyperparathyroidism in older adults as the key contributors to postmenopausal osteoporosis, but recent evidence has shown that numerous other pathophysiological mechanisms are involved in the onset of osteoporosis.

Recent studies have uncovered a novel interaction between the immune system and the skeletal system, known as osteoimmunology. The interaction between immune cells and bone cells—especially osteoclasts through common precursors with monocytes, macrophages, and dendritic cells can result in bone degradation in inflammatory conditions, such as periodontitis or rheumatoid arthritis [16]. In rheumatoid arthritis, the Th17 subset of CD4+ cells can activate osteoclasts to resorb bone in an osteoimmune disorder marked by bone erosions in various joints and synovial inflammation. These cells enhance bone resorption by the addition production of TNF and IL-6. A comparable process of the immune system is also observed in osteoporosis [17]. T-cells are thought to be an important source of pro-inflammatory cytokines; for example, postmenopausal women with osteoporosis exhibited the elevated levels of TNF-expressing cells and IL-17, generated by CD8+ and CD4+ T-cells. Recent studies on mice indicate that reduced estrogen levels lead to an increase in bone marrow dendritic cells, which produce IL-7 and IL-15. This leads memory T-cells to produce IL-17A and TNF, which subsequently results in bone resorption [18]. B-cells contribute to the pathophysiology of osteoporosis by generating RANKL and OPG, thereby serving as regulators, with their production rising in postmenopausal women [19]. Consequently, considerable evidence exists supporting the role of B-cells and T-cells in the progression of osteoporosis.

The diminish in ovarian activity and estrogen levels leads to bone loss during early menopause as estrogen receptors present on osteoblasts, osteoclasts, and osteocytes that directly influence their functions. Specifically, the loss of estrogen leads to an imbalance in the fundamental activity of the multicellular unit, promoting bone resorption by raising the count of osteoclasts while concurrently lowering the count of osteoblasts [20]. Estrogen deficiency contributes to bone loss by influencing bone cells directly as well as indirectly by enhancing inflammatory cytokines (TNF, IL-1, IL-6, and IL-17) [21].

Microorganisms in the gut that reside in the digestive system impact bone homeostasis, and the alteration of probiotics or antibiotics by gut micro-organisms influences bone health. Gut microbes have been demonstrated to impact the uptake of nutrients crucial for skeletal growth and consequently influence bone mineral density. Intestinal microorganisms generate short-chain fatty acids (SCFAs) following the fermentation of dietary fiber. SCFAs are linked to enhance calcium absorption, inhibit osteoclast differentiation, encourage Treg development, and restrain Th17 cells. Consequently, SCFAs play a crucial role in maintaining bone homeostasis.

Consequently, probiotics, gut microbes, and their metabolites could be a potential approach for preventing and treating osteoporosis [22].

Two main factors influence adult bone health: (i) achieving the highest level of peak bone mass (PBM) during growth and (ii) the speed of bone loss as one ages. Aging results in senescent cells (e.g., osteoblasts, osteocytes, and immune cells) within the bone microenvironment that releases pro-inflammatory SASP factors. Aging cells result in heightened bone resorption and diminished bone formation. Eliminating these cells or neutralizing them in mice has demonstrated decreased bone resorption and maintained bone formation. Significant advancements have been achieved in comprehending the influence of different mechanisms and elements that lead to bone loss [23].

4. Etiology

Bone mass normally peaks in young adults and then gradually declines, depending on genetic factors (such as vitamin D receptors), nutrition, weight-bearing activity, and hormonal levels. It appears that calcium intake in children and young adults is critical to the maintenance of bone mass later in life. Several factors predispose people to osteoporosis, including aging, decreased mobility or a sedentary lifestyle, hormonal factors, such as hyperparathyroidism, Cushing's syndrome, and continued intake of catabolic glucocorticoids such as prednisone. Prolonged intake of a diet deficient in calcium, vitamin D, or protein is associated with increased risk of osteoporosis. Other factors, such as a history of deficits in childhood or malabsorption disorders, cigarette smoking, and excessive caffeine intake, may also contribute to the development of osteoporosis [1].

5. Diagnosis and assessment

The diagnostic classification by the World Health Organization (WHO) is determined through bone mineral density (BMD) assessment using dual-energy X-ray absorptiometry (DXA), employing the T-score. This T-score is obtained by subtracting the mean BMD (in g/cm^2) of a young-adult reference group from the patient's BMD and then dividing the result by the standard deviation (SD) of the young-adult reference group. The International Society for Clinical Densitometry (ISCD) advises that bone mineral density (BMD) should be assessed at the lumbar spine (preferably L1–L4), total hip, and femoral neck. Osteoporosis cannot be diagnosed through BMD measurement at skeletal sites other than the lumbar spine, total hip, femoral neck, and 33% radius, or with methods other than DXA, except for total hip and femoral neck T-scores obtained from 2D projections of quantitative computed tomography (QCT) data [24, 25].

6. Nutrition in osteoporosis

Nutrition and physical activity are frequently used alongside pharmacological treatments for the prevention and management of osteoporosis. Nutrition is critical for skeletal wellness, in terms of reaching optimal BMD and in preserving bone mass; therefore, a well-balanced diet can prevent osteoporosis [26]. Certain nutrients are most frequently referenced in connection to BMD.

DOI: http://dx.doi.org/10.5772/intechopen.1012585

6.1 Macronutrient

6.1.1 Carbohydrate

It has been shown to have a positive effect on bone development and strength, as it is the primary energy source in the human body. They are found in fruits, grains, vegetables, and dairy products. They are found in foods as monosaccharides, disaccharides, oligosaccharides, and polysaccharides. Complex carbohydrates, specifically dietary fibers, are important for health and play a significant role in the prevention of osteoporosis [27].

Fiber is not broken down by human enzymes and thus is not digested or absorbed in the human body; it travels to the intestine, where gut microbes ferment it, generating short-chain fatty acids. These SCFAs enhance calcium absorption and have a beneficial effect on the bone, as stated previously [28]. Bakirhan et al. indicate that dietary fiber, and particularly soluble types, such as inulin, improves calcium absorption and BMD, especially in adolescents and postmenopausal females [29]. There is also some evidence that simple carbohydrates, such as refined (processed) sugar, in the diet may impact bone growth and strength; animal studies show that a high-glucose, high-sucrose diet decreases bone strength, affects osteoblast proliferation and differentiation, increases urinary calcium excretion, and inhibits calcium ion transport [30–33]. While carbohydrates play a critical role in blood glucose levels, poorly controlled diabetes is associated with increased bone fragility and hyperglycemia can compromise bone integrity, making diabetic bone disease a major health concern [34].

In conclusion, not every carbohydrate negatively impacts bone health. Specifically, complex carbohydrate sources can have positive effects, while simple or refined carbohydrate sources can have negative effects; therefore, reducing simple carbohydrates, like sucrose, glucose, or products made from refined flour, and increasing complex carbohydrates like cereals, fruits, and vegetables in the diet are important for improved bone health.

6.1.1.1 Summary

Choose carbs wisely:

- Not all carbs are harmful to bone health.
- *Complex carbohydrates* (e.g., from cereals, fruits, vegetables) are beneficial.
- *Simple/refined carbs* (e.g., sugar, white flour) may harm bones.
- Emphasis should be on reducing simple carbs and increasing complex carbs for stronger bones.

6.1.2 Protein

Dietary protein affects bones in several ways; it can be either beneficial or harmful, depending on the amount consumed (low-protein vs. high-protein diet) and its source (plant vs. animal). (a) Protein constitutes a significant part of the organic bone matrix, (b) regulates serum insulin-like growth factor 1 (IGF-1), and (c) might affect calcium metabolism. Proteins are also structural components of bone, accounting for 30% of bone mass and 50% of bone volume. Dietary protein also affects bone metabolism.

Observational studies indicate that increased protein intake correlates with higher BMD and may offer protective effects against bone loss, such as in the vertebral bone, among middle-aged and older adults. Proteins from animal sources (in eggs, meat, chicken, and dairy) are considered complete proteins (they contain all the essential amino acids) and are more nutritionally valuable than plant-based proteins.

Alanine, lysine, arginine, leucine, and glutamine stimulate insulin release that is required for osteoblasts to develop and differentiate. Lysine and arginine have been found to stimulate nitric oxide (NO) production and type I collagen formation, which could be used to prevent osteoporosis. Insufficient dietary protein can lead to muscle deterioration, which results in reduced bone mineral density (BMD) and a heightened risk of osteoporosis and fractures. Muscle mass enhances bone strength, while age-related muscle loss, known as sarcopenia, is closely linked to low bone mineral density and osteoporosis, especially in the elderly. Research indicates that individuals with low muscle mass are at a greater risk of developing osteoporosis. Bioactive peptides generated from dietary proteins during digestion have been recognized as the potential agents for bone protection. They influence bone health by controlling osteoblast function and inflammatory indicators. Collagen peptides, along with peptides sourced from dairy and seafood, have demonstrated potential in improving bone mineral density and reducing the risk of osteoporosis [35].

6.1.2.1 Summary

- The amount and source of protein being important for bone health.
- High-quality protein intake supports stronger bones and helps prevent osteoporosis.
- Insufficient protein can weaken muscles and bones.
- A balanced diet with a good mix of animal and plant proteins, especially those rich in essential amino acids and bioactive peptides, is key to promoting bone strength and reducing fracture risk.

6.1.3 Lipids

Dietary fats can also affect bone health. Recent research has demonstrated the considerable impact of lipids on bone mineral density (BMD) and the likelihood of fractures [36]. Increased intake of saturated fatty acids (SFAs) has been associated with lower bone mineral density and a heightened risk of fractures, particularly among postmenopausal women and older men [37]. Conversely, monounsaturated fatty acids (MUFAs), particularly those from olive oil, seem to positively impact BMD, due to their high levels of vitamin E and phenolic compounds [38].

The relationship between polyunsaturated fatty acids (PUFAs) and bone health is more complex. Different fatty acids produce varying effects, although overall PUFA consumption is associated with positive outcomes for bone health. Significantly, EPA and DHA (omega-3 fatty acids) and arachidonic acid (omega-6) combinations can positively impact BMD, and older adults who consume more α-linolenic acid have fewer hip fractures [39]. However, excess arachidonic acid, an omega-6 fatty acid, combined with insufficient omega-3 s can negatively impact BMD. In fact, high intakes of n-3 PUFAs from fish and fish oil supplements protect against bone loss, particularly in women and the elderly. However, excess lipid consumption can also adversely affect bone health by inducing hyperinsulinemia, reducing calcium absorption, increasing bone resorption, and disrupting bone formation mechanisms, especially when high lipid consumption replaces other nutrients of equal caloric value [40].

Consequently, dietary fats have both positive and negative impacts on bone health based on their kind, consumption amount, and interaction with other nutrients. A well-balanced diet, specifically highlighting MUFAs and omega-3 PUFAs, along with lifestyle changes, is crucial for sustaining optimal bone health. In middle age, consuming seafood and foods high in omega-3 can aid in maintaining bone mineral density and reduce the likelihood of fractures.

6.1.3.1 Summary

- Dietary fats have both beneficial and harmful effects on bone health, depending on the type and amount consumed.

- Excess saturated fats can weaken bones, whereas MUFAs (like those in olive oil) and omega-3 PUFAs (from fish and seafood) support strong bones and reduce fracture risk.

- Therefore, especially in middle-aged and older adults, it is important to consume a balanced diet rich in healthy fats, particularly omega-3 s and MUFAs, while limiting saturated and excessive total fat intake.

6.2 Micronutrients

Essential vitamins and minerals, known as micronutrients, are necessary for promoting healthy bone development, preventing different illnesses, and ensuring overall physiological well-being. Except for vitamin D, which can be produced internally, all other micronutrients need to be obtained from food [41]. Calcium and vitamin D are the most thoroughly researched for their effectiveness in preventing and treating osteoporosis. Additional nutrients such as phosphorus, magnesium, zinc, selenium, and vitamins, are crucial for bone metabolism.

6.2.1 Minerals

6.2.1.1 Calcium

Calcium is essential not just for bone health but also as a crucial nutrient for managing neuromuscular functions, immune system responses, heart rate control, and multiple other bodily processes. Approximately 99% of the entire calcium in the human body is located in the bones, mainly as hydroxyapatite [42, 43]. Nutrition is important for normal bone growth and mineralization. Bone is constantly being reshaped through the coordinated activities of osteoclast-mediated bone resorption and osteoblast-mediated bone formation, with calcium balance being a major factor in this process. When calcium consumption is adequate or its uptake is hindered, the body adjusts by elevating parathyroid hormone (PTH) levels to release calcium from the bones to maintain serum calcium levels [44, 45]. The released PTH subsequently boosts osteoclast activity, resulting in bone resorption and, consequently, bone loss.

On the other hand, calcium deficiency can cause hormonal disturbances, accelerating age-related bone deterioration and elevate the risk of osteoporosis. Numerous studies consistently support a positive correlation between adequate calcium intake across the lifespan and increased bone mineral density (BMD) along with lower incidence of fractures [44, 46, 47]. However, calcium supplementation is only prescribed to individuals who are at risk of inadequate intake, decreased absorption, deficiency due to possible adverse outcomes, such as nephrolithiasis, or other heart problems [48–50]. This is supported by the meta-analysis by Tai et al. [51] that demonstrated lower clinical benefits of calcium supplementation alone for BMD (0.7–1.8%). According to Indian council of medical research (ICMR) and National institute of nutrition (NIN) 2020, the daily calcium requirement varies across life stages. Considering physiological demands, adults need 1000 mg/d, adolescents require 850–1050 mg/day, and increased intake is advised for postmenopausal and lactating women around 1000–2000 mg/day [52].

Milk and dairy items serve as the main dietary sources of calcium (Ca); however, significant quantities can also be found in foods such as salmon, almonds, leafy vegetables, legumes, tofu, seafood, and calcium-enriched products [26, 53]. Heaney's study indicates that calcium from calcium-fortified mineral waters is absorbed somewhat more effectively than calcium from milk [54]. Eating foods with low oxalic acid and those processed to decrease phytic acid through methods such as soaking, fermentation, germination, or enzymatic treatment can enhance calcium deposition in bones since they interfere with calcium absorption, rendering calcium-rich foods that contain them as ineffective sources of calcium [26]. Excess sodium in the diet increases calcium loss in the urine because both nutrients compete for reabsorption in the kidneys, whereas vitamin D and phosphorus increase calcium absorption [43]. Thus, maintaining the optimal calcium-to-phosphorus ratio of 1–2:1 is crucial for bone development [55]. The combination of calcium and vitamin D supplementation is proven to prevent bone loss, reduce bone turnover, and reduce the risk of nonspine fractures in postmenopausal women [46]. Block et al. [56] found that meals rich in protein (45 g protein) are linked to higher urinary calcium excretion and reduced calcium reabsorption by the kidneys. A different study involving 24-hour urine collection revealed that incorporating sulfur amino acids into a 50 g/day protein diet resulted in a 43% rise in urinary calcium, which was still significantly lower than the levels seen with a 150 g/day protein intake [57].

6.2.1.1.1 Summary

- Calcium is an essential nutrient for enduring bone health and general physiological function.
- Its efficacy relies not only on consumption but also on absorption, nutrient interactions, and lifestyle factors.
- Although obtaining calcium from food is the best and safest method to fulfil daily requirements, supplements can be beneficial for at-risk individuals when taken carefully.

6.2.1.2 Phosphorus

Phosphorus is essential for numerous cellular functions, as it is a key component of genetic material, high-energy phosphate compounds, and membrane phospholipids that facilitate energy transfer and signaling pathways. [58, 59]. It is the second most abundant mineral in the bone, with total body reserves ranging from 550 to 770 g, of which approximately 85% is present in bones and teeth as hydroxyapatite and phosphoproteins [60]. Although a phosphorus deficiency can cause stunted growth and rickets in children or osteomalacia in adults, such deficiencies are uncommon due to its high bioavailability and frequent food sources [61].

As per the Indian Council of Medical Research (ICMR) and National Institute of Nutrition (NIN) 2020, the Recommended Dietary Allowance (RDA) for phosphorus changes at various life stages to meet the physiological needs of growth, maintenance, and reproduction [52]. The RDA is 100 mg/day for ages 0–6 months and 275 mg/day for 7–12 months old. In early childhood, the need rises to 390 mg/day for kids aged 1–3 years, 540 mg/day for aged 4–6 years, and 600 mg/day for 7–9 years. During adolescence, the RDA increases considerably because of fast skeletal development. Children aged 10–12 need 720 mg/day, whereas those aged 13–15 need 1050 mg/day. This rises additionally to 1120 mg/day for both males and females aged 16–17 years. For adults, the daily phosphorus needs remain constant at 600 mg for both genders. Increased physiological demands during pregnancy and lactation elevate the RDA to 1200 mg/day for women who are pregnant and 1000 mg/day for those who are nursing [52].

In general, dietary deficiencies are rare, as phosphorus is abundant in Indian diets, particularly from cereals, legumes, dairy products, and animal products. When calcium and phosphorus intake are sufficient, Lee and Cho [61] report that increased phosphorus intake was associated with significant improvements in bone health: a 4.2% increase in BMC, a 2.1% increase in BMD, and a 45% reduction in risk of osteoporosis. Conversely, research from several animal studies has shown that high phosphorus consumption, especially with low calcium in the diet, can adversely affect bone density. This phenomenon is believed to be influenced by raised levels of parathyroid hormone (PTH) and heightened excretion of osteopontin (OPN), a crucial protein in the bone matrix involved in bone remodeling and mineralization [59, 62, 63]. Some research suggests that a high intake of phosphorus, especially from inorganic phosphate additives in drinks like cola, may adversely affect bone metabolism, particularly in adolescents and women after menopause [64, 65].

Nevertheless, a study by Kovacova et al. [66] showed no notable alterations in the microarchitecture of cortical or trabecular bone in adult mice after extended cola intake, as evaluated by micro-computed tomography. This absence of negative effects was probably due to the animals' well-rounded diet and adequate amounts of exercise. Cola, as one of the most frequently consumed drinks nowadays, includes phosphoric acid, which the body easily absorbs. Regular consumption might lower milk consumption, which could result in a reduced calcium intake and an increased intake of inorganic phosphorus. This change in eating habits can upset the balance between calcium and phosphorus. Based on the existing scientific knowledge, it is recommended to limit the intake of phosphate-containing additives to promote optimal bone health [67].

6.2.1.2.1 Summary

- Sufficient phosphorus consumption aids in bone mineralization and density, but excessive intake, particularly from processed foods containing phosphate additives, can disturb the calcium-phosphorus equilibrium, potentially resulting in negative bone effects.

- Maintaining a balanced calcium-to-phosphorus ratio is important for optimal bone health.

- A well-balanced, whole-food-focused diet continues to be essential for maintaining both bone health and general wellness.

6.2.1.3 Magnesium

Magnesium (Mg) is a micronutrient that is involved in a variety of metabolic, enzymatic, and structural functions in the body, including the formation of a complex with adenosine triphosphate (ATP) for cellular energy production, cofactor for more than 300 enzymatic reactions, structural component of cell membranes, and regulator of ion transport (antagonist of $Ca2+$ and $K+$). These enzymes are essential for the production of proteins, carbohydrates, nucleic acids, and other important biomolecules, as well as for supporting neuromuscular excitability and transmission [68]. Magnesium is an essential cofactor for a wide variety of physiological functions, including the structural stability of cell membranes, and regulation of ion transport, and acts as a natural antagonist to calcium ($Ca2+$) and potassium ($K+$).

A lack of magnesium can hinder the absorption and balance of these ions, potentially causing hypokalemia and hypocalcemia [69]. About 60% of magnesium in the body is located in bones, 20–30% in muscles, and the rest is found in soft tissues and extracellular fluids [70]. Importantly, one-third of skeletal magnesium is found within cortical bone, intimately linked to hydroxyapatite crystals and the matrix around it [71]. Magnesium is crucial for the formation and restructuring of bones. It promotes osteoblast growth, boosts alkaline phosphatase function, and aids in the mineralization process. At the same time, magnesium inhibits osteoclast-driven bone resorption, preserving skeletal equilibrium [72].

Bone metabolism can also be directly and indirectly disturbed in cases of magnesium deficiency: Increased osteoclastic activity, decreased osteoblastic function, altered vitamin D metabolism, and increased parathyroid hormone (PTH) secretion can all contribute to bone loss and decreased bone quality [70]. Research on animals has shown that a lack of magnesium leads to a decrease in bone mass, a reduction in mechanical strength of bones, deterioration of trabecular microarchitecture, and thinning of cortical bone [73, 74]. Likewise, clinical research indicates that low dietary magnesium is linked to reduced bone mineral density (BMD), especially in women after menopause. Orchard et al. [75] noted diminished total body and hip BMD in women with lower magnesium consumption, although no direct link between magnesium intake and fracture risk was confirmed.

The increase magnesium intake effects on bone health. Certain research, like Nieves and Orchard et al. [46, 75], observed that the possible rise in wrist fracture risk associated with higher magnesium consumption. These results also might be influenced by elevated physical activity levels among individuals with higher magnesium consumption. Interestingly, the same study also reported small but significant increases (2–3%) in whole-body and lumbar spine BMD in women consuming more than 422.5 mg of magnesium per day, compared with women taking less than 206.5 mg per day. In addition, Ilich et al. and Ryder et al. [76] found that magnesium intake, especially in combination with calcium, positively affected BMD in premenopausal and postmenopausal women.

Magnesium-rich foods include green leafy vegetables (spinach), legumes, seeds, nuts, whole grains, and seafood [68, 77]. According to the 2020 Indian Council of Medical Research (ICMR) and the National Institute of Nutrition (NIN), the RDA for magnesium is 440 mg/day for adult males and 370 mg/day for adult females. These are slightly higher than the needs for pregnant (440 mg/day) and breastfeeding women (400 mg/day), which reflect increased physiological needs during these life stages [52]. Many factors influence magnesium levels, including age, exercise, smoking, and pre-existing health conditions. Serum magnesium levels can decrease to 60–80% of the levels seen in younger individuals as people age [70].

Moreover, lack of physical activity, smoking, high consumption of alcohol and caffeine, along with chronic illnesses such as diabetes, heart diseases, and osteoporosis can greatly diminish skeletal magnesium levels [69, 78]. Frequent intake of magnesium-dense foods like seafood has been demonstrated to enhance skeletal magnesium levels [79]. Recent researches demonstrated the importance of sufficient magnesium consumption in preserving ideal bone health and for the prevention of osteoporosis. Additional randomized controlled trials are needed for more establishing therapeutic benefits.

6.2.1.3.1 Summary

- Magnesium aids in bone development, prevents bone breakdown, and preserves skeletal strength.

- A sufficient dietary intake of magnesium, particularly when combined with calcium, is advantageous for bone health, but too much intake or supplementation must be handled carefully.

- A well-balanced diet abundant in natural magnesium sources, such as leafy vegetables, nuts, and fish, combined with healthy lifestyle habits, is essential for maintaining bone strength and avoiding age-related bone deterioration.

6.2.2 Vitamins

6.2.2.1 Vitamin D

Vitamin D, a fat-soluble secosteroid, occurs mainly in two forms—ergocalciferol (D_2) from plant sources and supplements, and cholecalciferol (D_3), sourced from animal products and produced in the skin when exposed to ultraviolet B (UVB) rays. The skin's endogenous production accounts for about 80–90% of a person's overall vitamin D needs, with the rest needed from diet or supplements [80].

Both forms of vitamin D undergo two consecutive hydroxylation processes after entering the body: first in the liver, where they are converted to 25-hydroxyvitamin D [25(OH) D], and then in the kidneys, where they are converted to the active form 1,25-dihydroxyvitamin D [1,25(OH)2D or calcitriol] [81].

Calcitriol helps in the maintenance of calcium and phosphate balance, increases calcium uptake in the intestine, increases renal calcium reabsorption, and regulating parathyroid hormone (PTH) release [82]. Regarding skeletal health, vitamin D plays both direct and indirect roles. It aids in bone mineralization and muscle performance, thus lowering the likelihood of falls and fractures, particularly in older adults [83]. Sufficient vitamin D levels support the maintenance of serum calcium and phosphate levels that are crucial for the formation of the bone matrix [80]. The primary dietary sources of vitamin D consist of fatty fish (e.g., salmon, mackerel), egg yolk, cod liver oil, and fortified foods, such as cereals and dairy items. Dietary sources play an important part, but because of the lack of rich sources, supplementation is often needed, particularly for high-risk groups [84]. Serum concentrations of 25(OH) D are considered optimal at ≥20 ng/mL for the general population and ≥ 30 ng/mL for individuals who are at risk of bone loss or fractures [85]. Supplemental vitamin D, especially when used in combination with calcium, has been shown to improve bone density and reduce the incidence of fractures [86]. Also, findings from meta-analyses continue to be unclear concerning its independent impact on osteoporosis prevention [87, 88].

Burt et al. [89] noted that high doses of vitamin D supplementation in healthy adults could decrease bone mineral density (BMD) without necessarily compromising bone strength. Conversely, sufficient vitamin D levels show a positive correlation with trabecular bone score (TBS)—a non-direct assessment of bone microarchitecture—in adults who maintain adequate serum vitamin D concentrations [90]. This suggests that vitamin D is especially beneficial for individuals who have existing metabolic bone disorders, such as osteoporosis or long-term vitamin D deficiency, and it is considered more effective to use vitamin D and calcium supplements simultaneously for these conditions [91]. Beyond the skeleton, vitamin D has other functions, including modulating immune responses, controlling inflammation, and contributing to muscle health.

A lack of it has been associated with autoimmune disorders, infections, and long-term illnesses [92]. Notably, vitamin D deficiency significantly increases the risk of hip fractures, particularly in the elderly [93]. In one study, 50% of postmenopausal women with hip fractures were found to be vitamin D deficient [93]. There are a variety of factors that can reduce the absorption or bioavailability of vitamin D. Certain drugs, like orlistat, interfere with fat absorption and therefore can interfere with the absorption of vitamin D [94]. Excessive vitamin A intake has been shown to reduce vitamin D bioavailability by approximately 30% [95]. The prevalence of vitamin D deficiency is also high in the obese population, likely due to sequestration in adipose tissue, which results in lower circulating levels, and thus, they require larger doses to achieve adequacy [96]. Interestingly, vitamin D supplementation has been shown to be not only effective at correcting deficiency in obese individuals, but also to positively affect the management of complications related to obesity [97].

Although vitamin D toxicity is rare, it can occur with high doses; high intermittent doses (e.g., boluses over 100,000 IU) are associated with an increased risk for falls and fractures in the elderly [98]. The primary risk of vitamin D overdose is hypercalcemia, which remains a concern, especially with synthetic derivatives or high-dose administrations, which should be restricted to monitored clinical settings [99]. Still, consistent supplementation with physiological amounts of cholecalciferol (D $_3$) is typically safe and effective for preventing deficiency and promoting bone health.

6.2.2.1.1 Summary

- Vitamin D is an essential nutrient for bone health, mainly due to its involvement in calcium and phosphate metabolism, mineralization of bones, and muscle function.

- Sufficient levels aid in preventing osteoporosis, lowering fall risk, and enhancing bone density, especially when paired with calcium supplementation.

- Diet and sunlight are primary sources, in case of older adults, obese, and individuals on specific medications, supplements are needed to achieve adequate levels.

6.2.2.2 Vitamin K

Vitamin K is a fat-soluble vitamin essential for bone metabolism, blood clotting, and several metabolic processes. It is found in two forms: vitamin K1 (phylloquinone) and vitamin K2 (menaquinone). Phylloquinone is the primary form of vitamin K present in food like leafy greens such as kale, spinach, cabbage, broccoli, and cauliflower [100]. Menaquinones are the secondary form generated by gut microbiota and can be found in animal products and fermented foods, including cheese, eggs, liver, natto (fermented soybeans), meat, and dairy products [101].

As per the ICMR–NIN Expert Group (2020), the Recommended Dietary Allowance for vitamin K is 55 μg/day for adult males and female, consistent with FAO/WHO guidelines for developing nations [52]. Epidemiological research has found the association between low vitamin K consumption with an increased risk of bone weakness and fractures. Feskanich et al. reported an increased occurrence of hip fractures in both premenopausal and postmenopausal women with inadequate vitamin K intake [102].

Vitamin K plays key role in bone health by the management of osteocalcin, which is a non-collagenous protein produced by osteoblasts. This protein needs vitamin K for the γ-carboxylation process to effectively bind to hydroxyapatite in the bone matrix [103]. Carboxylatedosteocalcin aids in bone strength and mineralization, but the undercarboxylated variant has been recognized as a bioactive hormone affecting insulin secretion, glucose metabolism, muscle nutrient absorption, and also brain and fertility functions [104, 105].

In addition to bone, vitamin K is crucial for the production of coagulation factors II, VII, IX, and X. Its impact, however, also encompasses cardiovascular health. Vitamin K2, specifically, is linked to decreased arterial calcification and a reduced risk of coronary heart disease, whereas K1 seems to have a neutral or limited impact on cardiovascular results [106, 107]. Moreover, vitamin K levels might influence physical performance, although its relationship with muscle strength is still uncertain [108]. In relation to bone aging and osteoporosis, vitamin K2 demonstrates potential advantages. It participates in inhibiting osteoclastogenesis through the modulation of the RANK/RANKL/OPG pathway, an essential process in bone resorption. Furthermore, vitamin K2 enhances osteoblast function by activating the steroid and xenobiotic receptor (SXR), facilitating collagen production and bone matrix formation [109, 110].

Various clinical and animal trials have found the positive effects of menaquinone-7 (MK-7) by improving bone mineral density (BMD), especially at the lumbar spine, and prevents age-related bone loss. These effects are seen in those with osteoporosis or in postmenopausal women, as shown by Knapen et al. and Shiraki et al. [111, 112]. Nonetheless, these advantages were not seen in healthy individuals [113]. The combination of vitamin K2, calcium, and vitamin D3 has been shown to improve BMD and lower fracture risk more efficiently than supplementation with individual nutrients [114, 115]. This combination therapy could be beneficial for postmenopausal women and individual with osteoporosis.

Moreover, vitamin K can affect other postmenopausal treatments, such as vitamin E, estrogen replacement, calcium, and various hormones, impacting their effectiveness and safety in maintaining bone health [116]. These exchanges emphasize the significance of a tailored, balanced nutritional and therapeutic approach for preserving bone health in elderly groups.

6.2.2.2.1 Summary

- Vitamin K2 is essential for bone metabolism. Supplementing with vitamin K has demonstrated the beneficial for the weakened bone health.

- Combination of different nutrient such as vitamin K2 with calcium and vitamin D3 seems to be the more effective in preserving bone density and lowering fracture risk.

- Its relationships with other bone-supporting treatments highlight the necessity of a tailored and balanced nutritional strategy to enhance skeletal and general well-being, especially in older adults.

6.2.2.3 Vitamin C

Vitamin C (ascorbic acid) is a water-soluble vitamin essential for numerous physiological functions, including the production of collagen, L-carnitine, hydroxyproline, hydroxylysine, various hormones (such as noradrenaline/adrenaline, peptide hormones), gene transcription, translation control, and tyrosine removal, all of which rely on vitamin C [117, 118]. Vitamin C serves as an antioxidant and aids in preventing diseases linked to oxidative stress [119]. Regarding bone, it serves as an essential cofactor for collagen production, osteoblast formation and development, and the suppression of osteoclast differentiation [120].

Epidemiologic studies show that vitamin C deficiency is linked to poor collagen production, improper osteoid formation, increased bone loss, and a higher risk of fractures, especially at the femoral neck and total hip [121], recommending its therapeutic potential for osteoporosis treatment. Various studies have indicated the positive relationship between vitamin C consumption and bone mineral density (BMD), in which it enhances the gene expression for osteoblast differentiation, boosting osteoblast activity, and speeding up bone formation. These effects were not found in other researches; for example, the study by Ahmadieh and Arabi found no significant changes in BMD with vitamin C supplementation in postmenopausal women, highlighting the necessity for additional research [122]. Moreover, combination of vitamins C and E supplementation might have bone-protective effects similar to those gained from resistance training in older women.

As per National Institute of Nutrition (NIN), the dietary recommendation (RDA) for vitamin C is 90 mg/day for adult males and 75 mg/day for adult females [52]. This suggests the amount required to sustain nearly maximal neutrophil levels while minimizing urinary ascorbate excretion, offering antioxidant defense, as stated by the National Institutes of Health (NIH).

6.2.2.3.1 Summary

- Vitamin C is essential for bone health, mainly due to its involvement in collagen production and the regulation of cells that build and break down bone.

- Ideal intake of vitamin C, whether through food or specific supplements, continues to be an effective approach for preserving bone density and reducing fracture risk.

6.3 Phytonutrients

Oxidative stress is a significant risk factor for the bone loss and osteoporosis. It impairs the activities of bone cells like osteoblasts and osteoclasts, causing bone deterioration. Body uses both internal antioxidant (such as superoxide dismutase (SOD), glutathione peroxidase (GPx), and catalase) and external antioxidants from diet (such as lycopene and polyphenols, present in fruits and vegetables). When these defenses are strained, repair antioxidants (like DNA repair enzymes) attempt to mend the damage [123]. Lycopene decreases osteoclast differentiation, improves intercellular gap junction communication, lowers inflammatory cytokine expression, modulates cell proliferation and differentiation during bone cell remodeling, and boosts osteoblast differentiation [124].

The antioxidant and anti-inflammatory properties of polyphenols contribute to reducing the adverse effects of OP-induced disruptions in osteoclastogenesis and osteoblast development. Polyphenols might aid in preventing bone loss by promoting osteoclast apoptosis. Polyphenols may directly influence osteoclasts or indirectly stimulate the NF-Kb/RANKL/OPG pathway in bone marrow mesenchymal stem cells (BMSCs), although further research is needed. Polyphenols not only provide a restricted therapeutic benefit for osteoporosis but they also pose specific risks, so they cannot serve as a comprehensive solution [125].

6.3.1 Summary

- Antioxidants such as lycopene and polyphenols may counteract these effects by promoting bone cell health and minimizing inflammation.

- Although dietary antioxidants appear beneficial in preventing oxidative bone harm, they ought to be considered as components of a comprehensive prevention approach rather than as isolated treatments (**Table 1**).

Nutrient type	Bone health impact	Mechanisms/key notes	Recommendation
Carbohydrate	• Effects depend on the type of carbohydrates [7]		
Complex carbohydrates (dietary fiber)	• *Positive impact* on bone mineral density and calcium absorption	• Fermented to SCFAs in colon → ↑ calcium absorption	25–30 grams per day [Inulin: (≥8–10 g/day) improves BMD in adolescents and postmenopausal women] [126]
High glycemic index simple carbs (glucose, sucrose, refined carbs, SSBs)	• Lower bone strength • Reduced osteoblast activity • Increased urinary calcium loss	• Elevated insulin/glucose → hypercalciuria, inhibition of osteoblasts • Soda acid/phosphate disrupt calcium absorption	Less than 10% of total energy intake [127]
Protein	• Generally beneficial *if calcium intake is adequate* • Modest improvements in lumbar spine BMD	• Essential for bone matrix and stimulating IGF-1 • which promotes bone formation • High-protein intake may increase urinary calcium, but this often reflects enhanced absorption, not bone loss	1.0–1.2 g/kg/day [128]
Protein type	• Animal protein tends to show stronger association with BMD • Plant protein may be less effective unless calcium/vitamin D are adequate	• Animal protein provides complete amino acid profile and often comes with calcium/D vitamin • Plant protein benefits if diet balanced in other nutrients.	
Lipids	• Some saturated fats linked to lower BMD • Moderate MUFA and omega-3 PUFA intake may support BMD • High omega-6 or excessive fats might be harmful	• Higher saturated fat intake inversely associated with hip BMD • above which benefit appears • ω-3 PUFAs reduce inflammation and support osteogenesis; excess ω-6 may increase fracture risk	20–35% of total calories SFA less than 10% of daily calories MUFAs ~20 g/day [129]
Calcium and vitamin D	• Reduces bone loss and fracture risk, especially in older adults and postmenopausal women	• Calcium provides a structural mineral; 99% resides in bones • Vitamin D enhances intestinal calcium absorption, supports mineralization and muscle function; combined • Supplementation is more effective than either alone	Calcium: ~1000–1200 mg/day [52] Vitamin D: 600–800 IU or more if deficient [130]
Vitamin K	• Particularly vitamin K_2 shows promise in improving BMD and reducing bone loss in postmenopausal/osteoporotic individuals	• Critical cofactor for carboxylation of osteocalcin • Essential for bone mineralization • K_2 enhances osteoblast activity and suppresses osteoclastogenesis; synergistic effects with calcium and D_3	55 micrograms (mcg)/day [52]

Nutrient type	Bone health impact	Mechanisms/key notes	Recommendation
Magnesium	• Adequate intake supports BMD, osteoblast activity, and calcium utilization • Deficiency reduces bone quality and may impair vitamin D metabolism	• Cofactor for hundreds of enzymes • Supports mineralization and inhibits resorption • Deficiency strongly linked to low BMD in older women	370–440 mg/day [52]
Phosphorus	• Necessary in proper ratio with calcium • High phosphorus (especially from soft drinks) can impair bone if calcium is low	• Critical component of bone mineral • Imbalance with calcium (e.g. high inorganic P) raises PTH and bone • loss risk	Adults (19 years and older): 700 mg per day Adolescents (9–18 years): 1250 mg per day [128]
Vitamin C	• Supports collagen synthesis and osteoblast differentiation • Deficiency increases fracture risk; some epidemiologic studies show a positive association with BMD	• Required for collagen formation and antioxidant protection in bone tissue • Evidence is strongest when dietary, rather than supplemental	90 mg/day for adult men 75 mg/day for adult women [52]

Table 1.
Summary of different nutrients, its effect on bone health, and recommendation.

7. Effects of physical activity in osteoporosis

Osteoporosis is more likely in people who are not active, which can be changed. If people become more active at any point in their lives, it may be good for their bones, but if they become less active, they may lose bones. [131]. According to the research, a woman who has gone through menopause loses 1.5% of her spine's bone each year and 1.1–1.4% of her femoral neck's bone every year for the first 4–5 years.

Various studies have revealed that physical activity during adolescence has skeletal effects that last into early adulthood, whereas activity-associated bone loading during young adulthood boosts BMD in middle-aged and older adults. In addition to increasing BMD, bone loading in adulthood enhances bone growth, cortical area, and strength while decreasing the risk of fractures [132]. Adult skeletal health is maintained through a dynamic balance of bone production and resorption. Studies have shown that exercise and sports activities can provide mechanical stimulation to joint tissues and bone, which are required to preserve tissue characteristics. On the contrary, mechanical unloading causes a loss of bone mass and can even lead to osteoporosis [133].

Exercise can impact bone through a variety of ways, including muscular contraction forces, gravitational loads, and endocrine/paracrine responses. During physical activity, bone is subjected to mechanical forces generated by muscle contraction and gravity loading. At the molecular level, bone cells (osteocytes) detect mechanical stresses as cell deformation, variations in extracellular fluid shear stress, pressure gradients, and electric fields [134]. Physical activity is an important way to handle osteoporosis, especially for older adults. It puts more force on the bones as it works with hormones and immune system, which help build up the bones while reducing bone loss. This teamwork helps keep bones strong and dense over the years. In addition, weak blood vessel growth in the bone greatly adds to weak and unhealthy bones. Working out helps blood vessel growth by turning on important growth helpers and signal paths, leading to good bone rebuilding and food supply [135].

Several workouts have been identified to stimulate bone formation and preserve bone mass; the ideal interventions favor a mechanical stimulus on bone both through antigravity loading and the tension placed on muscles [136]. Generally, therapeutic exercises for osteoporosis can be divided into two types of activities:

1. Weight-bearing aerobic exercises include walking, stair climbing, jogging, volleyball, tennis, Tai Chi, and dance.

2. Strength/resistance exercises involve moving joints against resistance, such as free weights, machines, tubing, or body weight [137].

Exercise in the elderly and osteoporotic individuals must be carefully planned depending on muscular strength, balance, mobility, cardiovascular health, bone density, fracture history, and fall risk. High-impact workouts that are useful in youth may be threatening for this population. To avoid injury, programs in severe osteoporosis should progress gradually, with no trunk flexion or rotation allowed [137].

8. Recommendation for prevention of osteoporosis

- Few guidelines have been recommended for the prevention of osteoporosis. One of them is Biver et al. [130], which states that the Mediterranean diet is associated with better bone health; therefore, it can be recommended for the prevention of osteoporosis.

- Vegetarian or vegan diets are associated with poorer bone health; therefore, they should be avoided or an adjustment of calcium intake should be systematically proposed.

- In overweight and obese patients, weight loss is recommended with regular, suitable weight-bearing physical activity, combined with the sufficient levels of vitamin D and calcium intake, to prevent the bone loss caused by restricted calorie intake.

- Optimal protein intake is important for the prevention of osteoporosis, a protein intake of at least 1–1.2 g/kg/day as part of a balanced diet with adequate amount of calorie, calcium, and vitamin D is recommended.

- Protein with high biological value, such as animal and dairy sources, should be included.

- The literature shows that the consumption of dairy products has a beneficial effect on BMD and is associated with a decreased fracture risk. Fermented dairy products (yoghurt, cheese) have a more beneficial effect on fracture risk. Consumption of two to three different dairy products a day is recommended to prevent osteoporosis.

- Recommended dietary calcium intake should be approximately 1 g/day. Along with calcium, vitamin D should be included in the diet.
- In case of vitamin D deficiency, supplementation should be preferred over dietary sources to maintain the vitamin D status.
- Daily soda consumption harms bone health. Therefore, restriction of soda beverages is recommended.
- Light-to-moderate alcohol consumption seems to have no adverse effect on bone health in women. On the other hand, heavy consumption is associated with lower BMD values and higher fracture risk. However, since alcohol is addictive and detrimental to health in general, alcohol consumption, even in moderation, is not recommended.
- Prebiotics, which form the substrate for our bacterial microflora, have a modest beneficial effect on intestinal calcium absorption. Although some probiotic strains have been reported to be associated with a modest reduction in bone loss, these can be recommended for the prevention of osteoporosis.

8.1 Summary

Osteoporosis is an increasing health concern worldwide and can cause serious threats to life. Therefore, focusing on preserving bone health and reducing the risk of osteoporosis are essential. Nutritional therapy have been found to be essential for both preventing and treating osteoporosis. Dietary changes and sufficient supplementation at different stages of life is vital to avoid nutrient deficiencies that could lead to the onset of osteoporosis. Both macronutrients and micronutrients serve distinct roles that influence bone health. The type, quantity, and various sources of nutrients can either have beneficial or detrimental effects. The essential nutrients for supporting the skeletal system include protein, complex carbohydrates, fiber, calcium, magnesium, phosphorus, and vitamins D, K, and C. The regular consumption of these nutrients in the diet increases the effectiveness of treatment and helps in the prevention of osteoporosis. Along with dietary modification, lifestyle changes are also required such as increasing physical activity and limiting alcohol or carbonated drink intake. Therefore, adopting a healthy lifestyle with a balanced diet and regular exercise can improve bone metabolism and overall bone health.

Author details

Samiya Khan[1,2*], Bhagyashree Parab[1,2] and Sadaf Hasan[1,2]

1 Tata Memorial Hospital, Mumbai, India

2 Advanced Center for Treatment, Research and Education in Cancer, Mumbai, India

*Address all correspondence to: samiyakhan1508@yahoo.in

References

[1] Gould BE, Dyer R. Pathophysiology for the Health Professions. 4th ed. Saunders/Elsevier; 2011

[2] Harvey NC, Cooper C, editors. Osteoporosis: A Lifecourse Epidemiology Approach to Skeletal Health. CRC Press/Taylor & Francis Group; 2018

[3] Rosen CJ. The Epidemiology and Pathogenesis of Osteoporosis. MaineHealth Maine Medical Center; 2014. p. 640. Available from: https://knowledgeconnection.mainehealth.org/mmc/640

[4] NIH Consensus Development Panel on Osteoporosis Prevention, Diagnosis, and Therapy. Osteoporosis prevention, diagnosis, and therapy. JAMA. 2001;**285**(6):785-795. DOI: 10.1001/jama.285.6.785

[5] Aibar-Almazán A, Voltes-Martínez A, Castellote-Caballero Y, Afanador-Restrepo DF, Carcelén-Fraile MDC, López-Ruiz E. Current status of the diagnosis and management of osteoporosis. International Journal of Molecular Sciences. 2022;**23**(16):9465. DOI: 10.3390/ijms23169465

[6] Salari N, Darvishi N, Bartina Y, Larti M, Kiaei A, Hemmati M, et al. Global prevalence of osteoporosis among the world older adults: A comprehensive systematic review and meta-analysis. Journal of Orthopaedic Surgery and Research. 2021;**16**(1):669. DOI: 10.1186/s13018-021-02821-8

[7] Kanis JA, Cooper C, Rizzoli R, Reginster JY, Scientific Advisory Board of the European Society for Clinical and Economic Aspects of Osteoporosis (ESCEO) and the Committees of Scientific Advisors and National Societies of the International Osteoporosis Foundation (IOF). European guidance for the diagnosis and management of osteoporosis in postmenopausal women. Osteoporosis International: A Journal Established as Result of Cooperation between the European Foundation for Osteoporosis and the National Osteoporosis Foundation of the USA. 2019;**30**(1):3-44. DOI: 10.1007/s00198-018-4704-5

[8] Bijelic R, Milicevic S, Balaban J. Risk factors for osteoporosis in postmenopausal women. Medical Archives (Sarajevo, Bosnia and Herzegovina). 2017;**71**(1):25-28. DOI: 10.5455/medarh.2017.71.25-28

[9] Hanafy NM, Elsehaimy LA, Alzokm SM, Abd El-Raheem SI. Bone mineral density and risk factors of osteoporosis in children. The Egyptian Rheumatologist. 2022;**44**(3):257-260. ISSN 1110-1164. DOI: 10.1016/j.ejr.2022.01.003

[10] Kirazlı Y, Atamaz Çalış F, El Ö, Gökçe Kutsal Y, Peker Ö, Sindel D, et al. Updated approach for the management of osteoporosis in Turkey: A consensus report. Archives of Osteoporosis. 2020;**15**(1):137. DOI: 10.1007/s11657-020-00799-0

[11] Ponzetti M, Rucci N. Updates on osteoimmunology: What's new on the cross-talk between bone and immune system. Frontiers in Endocrinology. 2019;**10**:236. DOI: 10.3389/fendo.2019.00236

[12] Nakashima T, Hayashi M, Fukunaga T, Kurata K, Oh-Hora M, Feng JQ, et al. Evidence for osteocyte regulation of bone homeostasis through RANKL expression.

Nature Medicine. 2011;**17**(10):1231-1234. DOI: 10.1038/nm.2452

[13] Lin GL, Hankenson KD. Integration of BMP, Wnt, and notch signaling pathways in osteoblast differentiation. Journal of Cellular Biochemistry. 2011;**112**(12):3491-3501. DOI: 10.1002/jcb.23287

[14] Tsourdi E, Jähn K, Rauner M, Busse B, Bonewald LF. Physiological and pathological osteocytic osteolysis. Journal of Musculoskeletal & Neuronal Interactions. 2018;**18**(3):292-303

[15] Liang B, Burley G, Lin S, Shi YC. Osteoporosis pathogenesis and treatment: Existing and emerging avenues. Cellular & Molecular Biology Letters. 2022;**27**(1):72. DOI: 10.1186/s11658-022-00371-3

[16] Horton JE, Raisz LG, Simmons HA, Oppenheim JJ, Mergenhagen SE. Bone resorbing activity in supernatant fluid from cultured human peripheral blood leukocytes. Science (New York, N.Y.). 1972;**177**(4051):793-795. DOI: 10.1126/science.177.4051.793

[17] Tsukasaki M, Takayanagi H. Osteoimmunology: Evolving concepts in bone-immune interactions in health and disease. Nature Reviews. Immunology. 2019;**19**(10):626-642. DOI: 10.1038/s41577-019-0178-8

[18] Zhao R, Wang X, Feng F. Upregulated cellular expression of IL-17 by CD4+ T-cells in osteoporotic postmenopausal women. Annals of Nutrition & Metabolism. 2016;**68**(2):113-118. DOI: 10.1159/000443531

[19] Onal M, Xiong J, Chen X, Thostenson JD, Almeida M, Manolagas SC, et al. Receptor activator of nuclear factor κB ligand (RANKL) protein expression by B lymphocytes contributes to ovariectomy-induced bone loss. The Journal of Biological Chemistry. 2012;**287**(35):29851-29860. DOI: 10.1074/jbc.M112.377945

[20] Clarke BL, Khosla S. Physiology of bone loss. Radiologic Clinics of North America. 2010;**48**(3):483-495. DOI: 10.1016/j.rcl.2010.02.014

[21] Pacifici R, Rifas L, McCracken R, Avioli LV. The role of interleukin-1 in postmenopausal bone loss. Experimental Gerontology. 1990;**25**(3-4):309-316. DOI: 10.1016/0531-5565(90)90067-c

[22] Yu M, Malik Tyagi A, Li JY, Adams J, Denning TL, Weitzmann MN, et al. PTH induces bone loss via microbial-dependent expansion of intestinal TNF+ T cells and Th17 cells. Nature Communications. 2020;**11**(1):468. DOI: 10.1038/s41467-019-14148-4

[23] Farr JN, Xu M, Weivoda MM, Monroe DG, Fraser DG, Onken JL, et al. Targeting cellular senescence prevents age-related bone loss in mice. Nature Medicine. 2017;**23**(9):1072-1079. DOI: 10.1038/nm.4385

[24] Kanis JA. Assessment of fracture risk and its application to screening for postmenopausal osteoporosis: Synopsis of a WHO report. WHO study group. Osteoporosis International: A Journal Established as Result of Cooperation between the European Foundation for Osteoporosis and the National Osteoporosis Foundation of the USA. 1994;**4**(6):368-381. DOI: 10.1007/BF01622200

[25] Shuhart CR, Yeap SS, Anderson PA, Jankowski LG, Lewiecki EM, Morse LR, et al. Executive summary of the 2019 ISCD position development conference on monitoring treatment, DXA cross-calibration and least significant change, spinal cord injury, peri-prosthetic and

orthopedic bone health, transgender medicine, and pediatrics. Journal of Clinical Densitometry: The Official Journal of the International Society for Clinical Densitometry. 2019;**22**(4):453-471. DOI: 10.1016/j.jocd.2019.07.001

[26] Karpouzos A, Diamantis E, Farmaki P, Savvanis S, Troupis T. Nutritional aspects of bone health and fracture healing. Journal of Osteoporosis. 2017;**2017**:4218472. DOI: 10.1155/2017/4218472

[27] Zhang L, Zhao L, Xiao X, Zhang X, He L, Zhang Q. Association of dietary carbohydrate and fiber ratio with postmenopausal bone mineral density and prevalence of osteoporosis: A cross-sectional study. PLoS One. 2024;**19**(2):e0297332. DOI: 10.1371/journal.pone.0297332

[28] Soliman GA. Dietary fiber, atherosclerosis, and cardiovascular disease. Nutrients. 2019;**11**(5):1155. DOI: 10.3390/nu11051155

[29] Bakirhan H, Karabudak E. Effects of inulin on calcium metabolism and bone health. International Journal for Vitamin and Nutrition Research. Internationale Zeitschrift fur Vitamin- und Ernahrungsforschung. Journal International de Vitaminologie et de Nutrition. 2023;**93**(1):85-96. DOI: 10.1024/0300-9831/a000700

[30] Tjäderhane L, Larmas M. A high sucrose diet decreases the mechanical strength of bones in growing rats. The Journal of Nutrition. 1998;**128**(10):1807-1810. DOI: 10.1093/jn/128.10.1807

[31] Terada M, Inaba M, Yano Y, Hasuma T, Nishizawa Y, Morii H, et al. Growth-inhibitory effect of a high glucose concentration on osteoblast-like cells. Bone. 1998;**22**(1):17-23. DOI: 10.1016/s8756-3282(97)00220-2

[32] Ericsson Y, Angmar-Månsson B, Flores M. Urinary mineral ion loss after sugar ingestion. Bone and Mineral. 1990;**9**(3):233-237. DOI: 10.1016/0169-6009(90)90041-d

[33] Douard V, Sabbagh Y, Lee J, Patel C, Kemp FW, Bogden JD, et al. Excessive fructose intake causes 1,25-(OH)(2) D(3)-dependent inhibition of intestinal and renal calcium transport in growing rats. American Journal of Physiology. Endocrinology and Metabolism. 2013;**304**(12):E1303-E1313. DOI: 10.1152/ajpendo.00582.2012

[34] Turcotte AF, O'Connor S, Morin SN, Gibbs JC, Willie BM, Jean S, et al. Association between obesity and risk of fracture, bone mineral density and bone quality in adults: A systematic review and meta-analysis. PLoS One. 2021;**16**(6):e0252487. DOI: 10.1371/journal.pone.0252487

[35] Martiniakova M, Babikova M, Mondockova V, Blahova J, Kovacova V, Omelka R. The role of macronutrients, micronutrients and flavonoid polyphenols in the prevention and treatment of osteoporosis. Nutrients. 2022;**14**(3):523. DOI: 10.3390/nu14030523

[36] Romero-Márquez JM, Varela-López A, Navarro-Hortal MD, Badillo-Carrasco A, Forbes-Hernández TY, Giampieri F, et al. Molecular interactions between dietary lipids and bone tissue during aging. International Journal of Molecular Sciences. 2021;**22**(12):6473. DOI: 10.3390/ijms22126473

[37] Orchard TS, Cauley JA, Frank GC, Neuhouser ML, Robinson JG, Snetselaar L, et al. Fatty acid consumption and risk of fracture in the women's health initiative. The American Journal of Clinical Nutrition. 2010;**92**(6):1452-1460. DOI: 10.3945/ajcn.2010.29955

[38] García-Martínez O, Rivas A, Ramos-Torrecillas J, De Luna-Bertos E, Ruiz C. The effect of olive oil on osteoporosis prevention. International Journal of Food Sciences and Nutrition. 2014;**65**(7):834-840. DOI: 10.3109/09637486.2014.931361

[39] Farina EK, Kiel DP, Roubenoff R, Schaefer EJ, Cupples LA, Tucker KL. Protective effects of fish intake and interactive effects of long-chain polyunsaturated fatty acid intakes on hip bone mineral density in older adults: The Framingham osteoporosis study. The American Journal of Clinical Nutrition. 2011;**93**(5):1142-1151. DOI: 10.3945/ajcn.110.005926

[40] Longo AB, Ward WE. PUFAs, bone mineral density, and fragility fracture: Findings from human studies. Advances in Nutrition (Bethesda, Md.). 2016;**7**(2):299-312. DOI: 10.3945/an.115.009472

[41] Kraemer K, de Pee S, Badham J. Evidence in multiple micronutrient nutrition: From history to science to effective programs. The Journal of Nutrition. 2012;**142**(1):138S-142S. DOI: 10.3945/jn.111.142414

[42] Hejazi J, Davoodi A, Khosravi M, Sedaghat M, Abedi V, Hosseinverdi S, et al. Nutrition and osteoporosis prevention and treatment. Biomedical Research and Therapy. 2020;**7**(4):3709-3720. DOI: 10.15419/bmrat.v7i4.598

[43] Lorincz C, Manske SL, Zernicke R. Bone health: Part 1, nutrition. Sports Health. 2009;**1**(3):253-260. DOI: 10.1177/1941738109334213

[44] Ratajczak AE, Rychter AM, Zawada A, Dobrowolska A, Krela-Kaźmierczak I. Nutrients in the prevention of osteoporosis in patients with inflammatory bowel diseases. Nutrients. 2020;**12**(6):1702. DOI: 10.3390/nu12061702

[45] Cashman KD. Calcium intake, calcium bioavailability and bone health. The British Journal of Nutrition. 2002;**87**(Suppl 2):S169-S177. DOI: 10.1079/BJNBJN/2002534

[46] Nieves JW. Osteoporosis: The role of micronutrients. The American Journal of Clinical Nutrition. 2005;**81**(5):1232S-1239S. DOI: 10.1093/ajcn/81.5.1232

[47] Winzenberg T, Shaw K, Fryer J, Jones G. Effects of calcium supplementation on bone density in healthy children: Meta-analysis of randomised controlled trials. BMJ (Clinical Research Edition). 2006;**333**(7572):775. DOI: 10.1136/bmj.38950.561400.55

[48] Cano A, Chedraui P, Goulis DG, Lopes P, Mishra G, Mueck A, et al. Calcium in the prevention of postmenopausal osteoporosis: EMAS clinical guide. Maturitas. 2018;**107**:7-12. DOI: 10.1016/j.maturitas.2017.10.004

[49] Celotti F, Bignamini A. Dietary calcium and mineral/vitamin supplementation: A controversial problem. The Journal of International Medical Research. 1999;**27**(1):1-14. DOI: 10.1177/030006059902700101

[50] Capozzi A, Scambia G, Lello S. Calcium, vitamin D, vitamin K2, and magnesium supplementation and skeletal health. Maturitas. 2020;**140**:55-63. DOI: 10.1016/j.maturitas.2020.05.020

[51] Tai V, Leung W, Grey A, Reid IR, Bolland MJ. Calcium intake and bone mineral density: Systematic review and meta-analysis. BMJ (Clinical Research Edition). 2015;**351**:h4183. DOI: 10.1136/bmj.h4183

[52] ICMR – National Institute of Nutrition. Nutrient Requirements for Indians: Recommended Dietary Allowances (RDA) and Estimated Average Requirements (EAR). 2020th ed. Indian Council of Medical Research; 2020. Available from: https://www.nin.res.in/rdabook/brief_note.pdf

[53] Price CT, Langford JR, Liporace FA. Essential nutrients for bone health and a review of their availability in the average north American diet. The Open Orthopaedics Journal. 2012;**6**:143-149. DOI: 10.2174/1874325001206010143

[54] Heaney RP. Calcium intake and disease prevention. Arquivosbrasileiros de Endocrinologia e Metabologia. 2006;**50**(4):685-693. DOI: 10.1590/s0004-27302006000400014

[55] Pastore SM, Gomes PC, Rostagno HS, Albino LFT, Calderano AA, Vellasco CR, et al. Calcium levels and calcium: Available phosphorus ratios in diets for white egg layers from 42 to 58 weeks of age. Revista Brasileira de Zootecnia. 2012;**41**(12):2424-2432

[56] Block GD, Wood RJ, Allen LH. A comparison of the effects of feeding sulfur amino acids and protein on urine calcium in man. The American Journal of Clinical Nutrition. 1980;**33**(10):2128-2136. DOI: 10.1093/ajcn/33.10.2128

[57] Zemel MB, Schuette SA, Hegsted M, Linkswiler HM. Role of the sulfur-containing amino acids in protein-induced hypercalciuria in men. The Journal of Nutrition. 1981;**111**(3):545-552. DOI: 10.1093/jn/111.3.545

[58] Vorland CJ, Stremke ER, Moorthi RN, Hill Gallant KM. Effects of excessive dietary phosphorus intake on bone health. Current Osteoporosis Reports. 2017;**15**(5):473-482. DOI: 10.1007/s11914-017-0398-4

[59] Ciosek Ż, Kot K, Kosik-Bogacka D, Łanocha-Arendarczyk N, Rotter I. The effects of calcium, magnesium, phosphorus, fluoride, and lead on bone tissue. Biomolecules. 2021;**11**(4):506. DOI: 10.3390/biom11040506

[60] Butusov MY, Jernelov A. Phosphorus. An Element That Could Have Been Called Lucifer. Vol. 9. New York, NY, USA: Springer; 2013. ISBN 978-1-4614-6802-8

[61] Lee AW, Cho SS. Association between phosphorus intake and bone health in the NHANES population. Nutrition Journal. 2015;**14**:28. DOI: 10.1186/s12937-015-0017-0

[62] Soetan KO, Olaiya CO, Oyewole OE. The importance of mineral elements for humans, domestic animals and plants—A review. African Journal of Food Science. 2010;**4**(5):200-222

[63] Koyama Y, Rittling SR, Tsuji K, Hino K, Salincarnboriboon R, Yano T, et al. Osteopontin deficiency suppresses high phosphate load-induced bone loss via specific modulation of osteoclasts. Endocrinology. 2006;**147**(6):3040-3049. DOI: 10.1210/en.2005-0671

[64] Tucker KL, Morita K, Qiao N, Hannan MT, Cupples LA, Kiel DP. Colas, but not other carbonated beverages, are associated with low bone mineral density in older women: The Framingham osteoporosis study. The American Journal of Clinical Nutrition. 2006;**84**(4):936-942. DOI: 10.1093/ajcn/84.4.936

[65] Wyshak G. Teenaged girls, carbonated beverage consumption, and bone fractures. Archives of Pediatrics and Adolescent Medicine. 2000;**154**(6):610-613. DOI: 10.1001/archpedi.154.6.610

[66] Kovacova V, Omelka R, Mondockova V, Londzin P, Conka J,

Meliskova V, et al. Long-term cola intake does not cause evident pathological alterations in the femoral bone microstructure: An animal study in adult mice. Nutrients. 2023;**15**(3):583. DOI: 10.3390/nu15030583

[67] Kristensen M, Jensen M, Kudsk J, Henriksen M, Mølgaard C. Short-term effects on bone turnover of replacing milk with cola beverages: A 10-day interventional study in young men. Osteoporosis International: A Journal Established as Result of Cooperation between the European Foundation for Osteoporosis and the National Osteoporosis Foundation of the USA. 2005;**16**(12):1803-1808. DOI: 10.1007/s00198-005-1935-z

[68] Volpe SL. Magnesium in disease prevention and overall health. Advances in Nutrition (Bethesda, Md.). 2013;**4**(3):378S-383S. DOI: 10.3945/an.112.003483

[69] Rosanoff A, Weaver CM, Rude RK. Suboptimal magnesium status in the United States: Are the health consequences underestimated? Nutrition Reviews. 2012;**70**(3):153-164. DOI: 10.1111/j.1753-4887.2011.00465.x

[70] Rude RK, Gruber HE. Magnesium deficiency and osteoporosis: Animal and human observations. The Journal of Nutritional Biochemistry. 2004;**15**(12):710-716. DOI: 10.1016/j.jnutbio.2004.08.001

[71] Castiglioni S, Cazzaniga A, Albisetti W, Maier JA. Magnesium and osteoporosis: Current state of knowledge and future research directions. Nutrients. 2013;**5**(8):3022-3033. DOI: 10.3390/nu5083022

[72] He LY, Zhang XM, Liu B, Tian Y, Ma WH. Effect of magnesium ion on human osteoblast activity. Brazilian Journal of Medical and Biological Research = Revista Brasileira de Pesquisas Medicas e Biologicas. 2016;**49**(7):e5257. DOI: 10.1590/1414-431X20165257

[73] Rude RK, Kirchen ME, Gruber HE, Meyer MH, Luck JS, Crawford DL. Magnesium deficiency-induced osteoporosis in the rat: Uncoupling of bone formation and bone resorption. Magnesium Research. 1999;**12**(4):257-267

[74] Orchard TS, Larson JC, Alghothani N, Bout-Tabaku S, Cauley JA, Chen Z, et al. Magnesium intake, bone mineral density, and fractures: Results from the women's health initiative observational study. The American Journal of Clinical Nutrition. 2014;**99**(4):926-933. DOI: 10.3945/ajcn.113.067488

[75] Nieves JW. Skeletal effects of nutrients and nutraceuticals, beyond calcium and vitamin D. Osteoporosis International: A Journal Established as Result of Cooperation between the European Foundation for Osteoporosis and the National Osteoporosis Foundation of the USA. 2013;**24**(3):771-786. DOI: 10.1007/s00198-012-2214-4

[76] Ryder KM, Shorr RI, Bush AJ, Kritchevsky SB, Harris T, Stone K, et al. Magnesium intake from food and supplements is associated with bone mineral density in healthy older white subjects. Journal of the American Geriatrics Society. 2005;**53**(11):1875-1880. DOI: 10.1111/j.1532-5415.2005.53561.x

[77] Office of Dietary Supplements. Magnesium: Fact Sheet for Health Professionals. National Institutes of Health; 2020. Available from: https://ods.od.nih.gov/factsheets/Magnesium-HealthProfessional/

[78] Zofková I, Nemcikova P, Matucha P. Trace elements and bone health. Clinical Chemistry and Laboratory Medicine. 2013;**51**(8):1555-1561. DOI: 10.1515/cclm-2012-0868

[79] Kim MH, Yeon JY, Choi MK, Bae YJ. Evaluation of magnesium intake and its relation with bone quality in healthy young Korean women. Biological Trace Element Research. 2011;**144**(1-3):109-117. DOI: 10.1007/s12011-011-9044-7

[80] Holick MF. Vitamin D deficiency. The New England Journal of Medicine. 2007;**357**(3):266-281. DOI: 10.1056/NEJMra070553

[81] DeLuca HF. Overview of general physiologic features and functions of vitamin D. The American Journal of Clinical Nutrition. 2004;**80**(6 Suppl):1689S-1696S. DOI: 10.1093/ajcn/80.6.1689S

[82] Bouillon R, Marcocci C, Carmeliet G, Bikle D, White JH, Dawson-Hughes B, et al. Skeletal and extraskeletal actions of vitamin D: Current evidence and outstanding questions. Endocrine Reviews. 2019;**40**(4):1109-1151. DOI: 10.1210/er.2018-00126

[83] Bischoff-Ferrari HA, Dietrich T, Orav EJ, Hu FB, Zhang Y, Karlson EW, et al. Higher 25-hydroxyvitamin D concentrations are associated with better lower-extremity function in both active and inactive persons aged > or =60 y. The American Journal of Clinical Nutrition. 2004;**80**(3):752-758. DOI: 10.1093/ajcn/80.3.752

[84] Mithal A, Wahl DA, Bonjour JP, Burckhardt P, Dawson-Hughes B, Eisman JA, et al. Global vitamin D status and determinants of hypovitaminosis D. Osteoporosis International: A Journal Established as Result of Cooperation between the European Foundation for Osteoporosis and the National Osteoporosis Foundation of the USA. 2009;**20**(11):1807-1820. DOI: 10.1007/s00198-009-0954-6

[85] Holick MF, Binkley NC, Bischoff-Ferrari HA, Gordon CM, Hanley DA, Heaney RP, et al. Evaluation, treatment, and prevention of vitamin D deficiency: An Endocrine Society clinical practice guideline. The Journal of Clinical Endocrinology and Metabolism. 2011;**96**(7):1911-1930. DOI: 10.1210/jc.2011-0385

[86] Weaver CM, Gordon CM, Janz KF, Kalkwarf HJ, Lappe JM, Lewis R, et al. The National Osteoporosis Foundation's position statement on peak bone mass development and lifestyle factors: A systematic review and implementation recommendations. Osteoporosis International: A Journal Established as Result of Cooperation between the European Foundation for Osteoporosis and the National Osteoporosis Foundation of the USA. 2016;**27**(4):1281-1386. DOI: 10.1007/s00198-015-3440-3

[87] Boonen S, Lips P, Bouillon R, Bischoff-Ferrari HA, Vanderschueren D, Haentjens P. Need for additional calcium to reduce the risk of hip fracture with vitamin d supplementation: Evidence from a comparative metaanalysis of randomized controlled trials. The Journal of Clinical Endocrinology and Metabolism. 2007;**92**(4):1415-1423. DOI: 10.1210/jc.2006-1404

[88] Bolland MJ, Grey A, Gamble GD, Reid IR. The effect of vitamin D supplementation on skeletal, vascular, or cancer outcomes: A trial sequential meta-analysis. The Lancet. Diabetes & Endocrinology. 2014;**2**(4):307-320. DOI: 10.1016/S2213-8587(13)70212-2

[89] Burt LA, Billington EO, Rose MS, Raymond DA, Hanley DA, Boyd SK.

Effect of high-dose vitamin D supplementation on volumetric bone density and bone strength: A randomized clinical trial. JAMA. 2019;**322**(8):736-745. DOI: 10.1001/jama.2019.11889

[90] Alwan A, Al Rassy N, Berro AJ, Rizkallah M, Matta J, Frenn F, et al. Vitamin D and trabecular bone score in a group of young Lebanese adults. Journal of Clinical Densitometry: The Official Journal of the International Society for Clinical Densitometry. 2018;**21**(3):453-458. DOI: 10.1016/j.jocd.2018.02.002

[91] Tang BM, Eslick GD, Nowson C, Smith C, Bensoussan A. Use of calcium or calcium in combination with vitamin D supplementation to prevent fractures and bone loss in people aged 50 years and older: A meta-analysis. Lancet (London, England). 2007;**370**(9588):657-666. DOI: 10.1016/S0140-6736(07)61342-7

[92] Aranow C. Vitamin D and the immune system. Journal of Investigative Medicine: The Official Publication of the American Federation for Clinical Research. 2011;**59**(6):881-886. DOI: 10.2310/JIM.0b013e31821b8755

[93] LeBoff MS, Kohlmeier L, Hurwitz S, Franklin J, Wright J, Glowacki J. Occult vitamin D deficiency in postmenopausal US women with acute hip fracture. JAMA. 1999;**281**(16):1505-1511. DOI: 10.1001/jama.281.16.1505

[94] McDuffie JR, Calis KA, Booth SL, Uwaifo GI, Yanovski JA. Effects of orlistat on fat-soluble vitamins in obese adolescents. Pharmacotherapy. 2002;**22**(7):814-822. DOI: 10.1592/phco.22.11.814.33627

[95] Johansson S, Melhus H. Vitamin A antagonizes calcium response to vitamin D in man. Journal of Bone and Mineral Research: The Official Journal of the American Society for Bone and Mineral Research. 2001;**16**(10):1899-1905. DOI: 10.1359/jbmr.2001.16.10.1899

[96] Wortsman J, Matsuoka LY, Chen TC, Lu Z, Holick MF. Decreased bioavailability of vitamin D in obesity. The American Journal of Clinical Nutrition. 2000;**72**(3):690-693. DOI: 10.1093/ajcn/72.3.690

[97] Migliaccio S, Di Nisio A, Mele C, Scappaticcio L, Savastano S, Colao A, et al. Obesity and hypovitaminosis D: Causality or casualty? International Journal of Obesity Supplements. 2019;**9**(1):20-31. DOI: 10.1038/s41367-019-0010-8

[98] Sanders KM, Stuart AL, Williamson EJ, Simpson JA, Kotowicz MA, Young D, et al. Annual high-dose oral vitamin D and falls and fractures in older women: A randomized controlled trial. JAMA. 2010;**303**(18):1815-1822. DOI: 10.1001/jama.2010.594

[99] Vieth R. Vitamin D toxicity, policy, and science. Journal of Bone and Mineral Research: The Official Journal of the American Society for Bone and Mineral Research. 2007;**22**(Suppl 2):V64-V68. DOI: 10.1359/jbmr.07s221

[100] Booth SL. Roles for vitamin K beyond coagulation. Annual Review of Nutrition. 2009;**29**:89-110. DOI: 10.1146/annurev-nutr-080508-141217

[101] Shea MK, Booth SL. Update on the role of vitamin K in skeletal health. Nutrition Reviews. 2008;**66**(10):549-557. DOI: 10.1111/j.1753-4887.2008.00106.x

[102] Feskanich D, Weber P, Willett WC, Rockett H, Booth SL, Colditz GA. Vitamin K intake and hip fractures in women: A prospective study. The American Journal of Clinical Nutrition. 1999;**69**(1):74-79. DOI: 10.1093/ajcn/69.1.74

[103] Koshihara Y, Hoshi K, Okawara R, Ishibashi H, Yamamoto S. Vitamin K stimulates osteoblastogenesis and inhibits osteoclastogenesis in human bone marrow cell culture. The Journal of Endocrinology. 2003;**176**(3):339-348. DOI: 10.1677/joe.0.1760339

[104] Lee NK, Sowa H, Hinoi E, Ferron M, Ahn JD, Confavreux C, et al. Endocrine regulation of energy metabolism by the skeleton. Cell. 2007;**130**(3):456-469. DOI: 10.1016/j.cell.2007.05.047

[105] Tencerova M, Okla M, Kassem M. Insulin signaling in bone marrow adipocytes. Current Osteoporosis Reports. 2019;**17**(6):446-454. DOI: 10.1007/s11914-019-00552-8

[106] Beulens JW, Booth SL, van den Heuvel EG, Stoecklin E, Baka A, Vermeer C. The role of menaquinones (vitamin K_2) in human health. The British Journal of Nutrition. 2013;**110**(8):1357-1368. DOI: 10.1017/S0007114513001013

[107] Gast GC, de Roos NM, Sluijs I, Bots ML, Beulens JW, Geleijnse JM, et al. A high menaquinone intake reduces the incidence of coronary heart disease. Nutrition, Metabolism, and Cardiovascular Diseases: NMCD. 2009;**19**(7):504-510. DOI: 10.1016/j.numecd.2008.10.004

[108] Azuma K, Ouchi Y, Inoue S. Vitamin K: Novel molecular mechanisms of action and its roles in osteoporosis. Geriatrics & Gerontology International. 2014;**14**(1):1-7. DOI: 10.1111/ggi.12060

[109] Iwamoto J, Takeda T, Ichimura S. Effect of combined administration of vitamin D3 and vitamin K2 on bone mineral density of the lumbar spine in postmenopausal women with osteoporosis. Journal of Orthopaedic Science: Official Journal of the Japanese Orthopaedic Association. 2000;**5**(6):546-551. DOI: 10.1007/s007760070003

[110] Yamaguchi M, Weitzmann MN. Vitamin K2 stimulates osteoblastogenesis and suppresses osteoclastogenesis by suppressing NF-κB activation. International Journal of Molecular Medicine. 2011;**27**(1):3-14. DOI: 10.3892/ijmm.2010.562

[111] Knapen MH, Schurgers LJ, Vermeer C. Vitamin K2 supplementation improves hip bone geometry and bone strength indices in postmenopausal women. Osteoporosis International: A Journal Established as Result of Cooperation between the European Foundation for Osteoporosis and the National Osteoporosis Foundation of the USA. 2007;**18**(7):963-972. DOI: 10.1007/s00198-007-0337-9

[112] Shiraki M, Shiraki Y, Aoki C, Miura M. Vitamin K2 (menatetrenone) effectively prevents fractures and sustains lumbar bone mineral density in osteoporosis. Journal of Bone and Mineral Research: The Official Journal of the American Society for Bone and Mineral Research. 2000;**15**(3):515-521. DOI: 10.1359/jbmr.2000.15.3.515

[113] Cockayne S, Adamson J, Lanham-New S, Shearer MJ, Gilbody S, Torgerson DJ. Vitamin K and the prevention of fractures: Systematic review and meta-analysis of randomized controlled trials. Archives of Internal Medicine. 2006;**166**(12):1256-1261. DOI: 10.1001/archinte.166.12.1256

[114] Kanellakis S, Moschonis G, Tenta R, Schaafsma A, van den Heuvel EG, Papaioannou N, et al. Changes in parameters of bone metabolism in postmenopausal women following a 12-month intervention period using

dairy products enriched with calcium, vitamin D, and phylloquinone (vitamin K(1)) or menaquinone-7 (vitamin K (2)): The postmenopausal health study II. Calcified Tissue International. 2012;**90**(4):251-262. DOI: 10.1007/s00223-012-9571-z

[115] Villa JKD, Mishima MDV, Brum MF, Pizziolo VR, Diaz-Muñoz G, Martino HSD, et al. Effect of vitamin K and calcium in bone loss in ovariectomized rats. Anais da Academia Brasileira de Ciencias. 2026;**97**(suppl 4):e20250214. DOI: 10.1590/0001-3765202520250214

[116] Booth SL. Vitamin K: Food composition and dietary intakes. Food & Nutrition Research. 2012;**56**. DOI: 10.3402/fnr.v56i0.5505

[117] Devaki SJ, Raveendran RL. Vitamin C: Sources, functions, sensing and analysis. In: Hamza A, editor. Vitamin C. London, UK: IntechOpen; 2017. pp. 1-25. DOI: 10.5772/intechopen.70162

[118] Doseděl M, Jirkovský E, Macáková K, Krčmová LK, Javorská L, Pourová J, et al. Vitamin C-sources, physiological role, kinetics, deficiency, use, toxicity, and determination. Nutrients. 2021;**13**(2):615. DOI: 10.3390/nu13020615

[119] Pehlivan FE. Vitamin C: An Antioxidant Agent. London, UK: IntechOpen; 2017. DOI: 10.5772/intechopen.69660

[120] Finck H, Hart AR, Jennings A, Welch AA. Is there a role for vitamin C in preventing osteoporosis and fractures? A review of the potential underlying mechanisms and current epidemiological evidence. Nutrition Research Reviews. 2014;**27**(2):268-283. DOI: 10.1017/S0954422414000195

[121] Aghajanian P, Hall S, Wongworawat MD, Mohan S. The roles and mechanisms of actions of vitamin C in bone: New developments. Journal of Bone and Mineral Research: The Official Journal of the American Society for Bone and Mineral Research. 2015;**30**(11):1945-1955. DOI: 10.1002/jbmr.2709

[122] Ahmadieh H, Arabi A. Vitamins and bone health: Beyond calcium and vitamin D. Nutrition Reviews. 2011;**69**(10):584-598. DOI: 10.1111/j.1753-4887.2011.00372.x

[123] Rao LG, Rao AV. Oxidative stress and antioxidants in the risk of osteoporosis — Role of phytochemical antioxidants lycopene and polyphenol-containing nutritional supplements. In: Phytochemicals - Isolation, Characterisation and Role in Human Health. London, UK: IntechOpen; 2015. DOI: 10.5772/60446

[124] Walallawita US, Wolber FM, Ziv-Gal A, Kruger MC, Heyes JA. Potential role of lycopene in the prevention of postmenopausal bone loss: Evidence from molecular to clinical studies. International Journal of Molecular Sciences. 2020;**21**(19):7119. DOI: 10.3390/ijms21197119

[125] Su Z, Yao B, Liu G, Fang J. Polyphenols as potential preventers of osteoporosis: A comprehensive review on antioxidant and anti-inflammatory effects, molecular mechanisms, and signal pathways in bone metabolism. The Journal of Nutritional Biochemistry. 2024;**123**:109488. DOI: 10.1016/j.jnutbio.2023.109488

[126] Kim Y, Jang KH, Lee EY, Cho Y, Kang SA, Ha WK, et al. The effect of chicory fructan fiber on calcium absorption and bone metabolism in Korean postmenopausal women. Nutritional Science. 2004;7:151-157

[127] Yan RR, Louie JCY. Sugar guidelines should be evidence-based and contain simple and easily actionable messages. Frontiers in Nutrition. 2023;**10**:1227377. DOI: 10.3389/fnut.2023.1227377

[128] Biver E, Herrou J, Larid G, Legrand MA, Gonnelli S, Annweiler C, et al. Dietary recommendations in the prevention and treatment of osteoporosis. Joint Bone Spine. 2023;**90**(3):105521. DOI: 10.1016/j.jbspin.2022.105521

[129] Liu AG, Ford NA, Hu FB, Zelman KM, Mozaffarian D, Kris-Etherton PM. A healthy approach to dietary fats: Understanding the science and taking action to reduce consumer confusion. Nutrition Journal. 2017;**16**(1):53. DOI: 10.1186/s12937-017-0271-4

[130] Demay MB, Pittas AG, Bikle DD, Diab DL, Kiely ME, Lazaretti-Castro M, et al. Vitamin D for the prevention of disease: An Endocrine Society clinical practice guideline. The Journal of Clinical Endocrinology and Metabolism. 2024;**109**(8):1907-1947. DOI: 10.1210/clinem/dgae290

[131] Nordström A, Olsson T, Nordström P. Bone gained from physical activity and lost through detraining: A longitudinal study in young males. Osteoporosis International: A Journal Established as Result of Cooperation between the European Foundation for Osteoporosis and the National Osteoporosis Foundation of the USA. 2005;**16**(7):835-841. DOI: 10.1007/s00198-004-1749-4

[132] Daly RM, Bass SL. Lifetime sport and leisure activity participation is associated with greater bone size, quality and strength in older men. Osteoporosis International: A Journal Established as Result of Cooperation between the European Foundation for Osteoporosis and the National Osteoporosis Foundation of the USA. 2006;**17**(8):1258-1267. DOI: 10.1007/s00198-006-0114-1

[133] Robling AG, Castillo AB, Turner CH. Biomechanical and molecular regulation of bone remodeling. Annual Review of Biomedical Engineering. 2006;**8**:455-498. DOI: 10.1146/annurev.bioeng.8.061505.095721

[134] Turner CH, Robling AG. Mechanisms by which exercise improves bone strength. Journal of Bone and Mineral Metabolism. 2005;**23**(Suppl):16-22. DOI: 10.1007/BF03026318

[135] Tong X, Chen X, Zhang S, Huang M, Shen X, Xu J, et al. The effect of exercise on the prevention of osteoporosis and bone angiogenesis. BioMed Research International. 2019;**2019**:8171897. DOI: 10.1155/2019/8171897

[136] Bonaiuti D, Arioli G, Diana G, Franchignoni F, Giustini A, Monticone M, et al. SIMFER rehabilitation treatment guidelines in postmenopausal and senile osteoporosis. Europa Medicophysica. 2005;**41**(4):315-337

[137] Benedetti MG, Furlini G, Zati A, Letizia Mauro G. The effectiveness of physical exercise on bone density in osteoporotic patients. BioMed Research International. 2018;**2018**:4840531. DOI: 10.1155/2018/4840531

Chapter 5

Screening and Treatment of Pancreatitis-Associated Osteoporosis: Importance and Clinical Applications

Xin-Ying Tang, Jia-Yun Chen, Yuan-Chen Wang, Jian-Feng Yang, Zhuan Liao and Wen-Bin Zou

Abstract

Pancreatitis, in both its acute and chronic forms, is a common gastrointestinal disorder with numerous complications, including pancreatitis-associated osteoporosis (PAO)—a condition increasingly recognized for its impact on quality of life. This review examines the relationship between pancreatitis and osteoporosis, emphasizing the need for early screening and individualized treatment. Drawing on recent research, we offer evidence-based recommendations to support bone health in affected patients and advocate for a comprehensive, personalized approach to improve clinical outcomes.

Keywords: pancreatitis, osteoporosis, screening, treatment, clinical applications

1. Introduction

Pancreatitis is the inflammation of the pancreas, which produces digestive enzymes and hormones. It mainly includes acute (AP), chronic (CP), and autoimmune (AIP) subtypes. Pancreatitis represents a substantial global health burden, with contemporary epidemiological studies reporting a combined annual incidence of 44.3 cases per 100,000 population (AP: 34.8, CP: 8.7, AIP: 0.8/100,000) [1]. Emerging clinical evidence highlights osteoporosis as a critical complication of pancreatitis, especially CP. The prevalence rates of osteoporosis reach 20.9–24.7% and osteopenia rates are 41.2% in CP patients, reflecting a two- to threefold increase over matched control groups [1, 2]. Particularly, AIP cohorts exhibit a markedly higher osteoporosis prevalence (30–40%) [3, 4], primarily attributable to prolonged glucocorticoid therapy, whereas AP survivors sustain a 35% elevated fracture risk within 5 years post-diagnosis [5, 6]. Patients with CP exhibit an annual decline in spinal bone mineral density (BMD) of up to 2.3% [1, 7], approximately three times higher than the rate of age-related bone loss in healthy individuals of the same age.

The pathogenesis of pancreatitis-associated osteoporosis (PAO) centers on metabolic dysregulation, where pancreatic exocrine insufficiency (PEI) (present in >80% of advanced CP [7] and 62% of severe AP [8]) drives vitamin D malabsorption and trabecular bone deterioration. Concurrently, CP-associated diabetes (45% prevalence [9]) and post-pancreatectomy metabolic acidosis synergistically amplify fracture risk (2.8-fold [10]) through adipokine-mediated osteoblast suppression. Chronic inflammation amplifies osteoclast activity via IL-6/TNF-α in CP/AP, while AIP patients suffer dual autoimmune bone erosion and steroid-induced osteoblast suppression (>3% BMD decline per year) [10, 11]. Iatrogenic interventions significantly exacerbate fracture susceptibility in CP patients: pancreatic resections amplify CP-associated fracture risk by 4.7-fold through vitamin D malabsorption and metabolic acidosis [10]. Meanwhile, spinal surgeries paradoxically induce *de novo* AP via postoperative systemic inflammatory cascades involving IL-6/TNF-α elevation [12].

Global disparities in osteoporosis screening persist, shaped by healthcare infrastructure inequities. While high-income countries achieve only 41.7% dual-energy X-ray absorptiometry (DXA) screening compliance among pancreatitis patients, 93% of medical centers in low- and middle-income countries (LMICs)—where 78% of global pancreatitis cases occur—lack DXA access entirely [13]. Diagnostic delays average 28 months, due to primary care recognition gaps affecting 62% of at-risk patients. Although calcaneal quantitative ultrasound (QUS) demonstrates 86% sensitivity for detecting osteopenia in CP cohorts, insufficient validation across ethnic populations limits its guideline adoption. Opportunistic computed tomography (CT) screening detects early trabecular microarchitecture changes missed by DXA in 68% of cases, yet standardization challenges and implementation barriers hinder its widespread clinical integration [14–16].

The therapeutic management of PAO needs to be individualized according to different subtypes. For CP, pancreatic enzyme replacement therapy (PERT) combined with high-dose vitamin D_3 (4000–6000 IU per day) and calcium (1200–1500 mg per day) can stabilize BMD [13, 14]. However, using PERT alone may not fully reverse metabolic sequelae, and targeted interventions are still required for problems, such as fibroblast growth factor 23 (FGF-23)-mediated bone mineralization disorders [7, 14, 17]. In AP, vitamin D supplementation and weight-bearing exercise can alleviate osteopenia. Nevertheless, the "metabolic memory" effect caused by continuously elevated pro-inflammatory factors requires the monitoring of bone turnover markers in severe or recurrent AP patients [7, 13]. For AIP, proactive bone protection measures should be taken simultaneously during glucocorticoid treatment. Denosumab or teriparatide can effectively counteract steroid-induced bone loss. Meanwhile, IgG4-related bone marrow infiltration (manifested as bone sclerosis or atypical fractures) may require a biopsy for a definite diagnosis to guide treatment adjustments [7, 18].

Precision screening and "metabolo-orthopedic" strategies integrating pathophysiology and resources are essential [7]. In the following text, we elaborate on the mechanism of PAO, the importance and clinical applications of its screening and treatment, and future research directions.

2. The pathogenesis of pancreatitis-associated osteoporosis

2.1 Acute pancreatitis and osteoporosis

AP is a sudden inflammatory condition of the pancreas characterized by autodigestion of pancreatic tissue due to premature activation of digestive enzymes.

Pancreatitis subtype	Pathogenic mechanisms
Acute pancreatitis (AP)	1. Systemic inflammatory response (release of pro-inflammatory cytokines, such as TNF-α and IL-6): Promotes osteoclast activation and bone resorption; 2. Prolonged immobilization: Reduces mechanical load and stimulates bone resorption; 3. Vitamin D deficiency: Impairs calcium absorption and bone mineralization, reducing bone mineral density (BMD); 4. Hormonal imbalance (IGF-1 inhibition): Has a negative impact on bone health.
Chronic pancreatitis (CP)	1. Pancreatic exocrine insufficiency (PEI): Causes malabsorption of fat-soluble vitamins (e.g., vitamin D) and calcium, impairing bone mineralization; 2. Chronic inflammation (elevated IL-1β and RANKL): Stimulates osteoclast formation and increases bone resorption; 3. Comorbid diabetes: Insulin deficiency and accumulation of advanced glycation end products (AGEs) exacerbate bone fragility; 4. Advanced lesions (e.g., progressive CP): Combined effects of chronic inflammation, malnutrition, and hormonal imbalance accelerate bone loss.
Autoimmune pancreatitis (AIP)	1. Glucocorticoid therapy: Inhibits osteoblast activity, enhances osteoclast survival, and impairs intestinal calcium absorption, leading to rapid and severe bone loss; 2. Systemic inflammation (elevated TNF-α and IL-6): Promotes osteoclast activation; 3. IgG4-mediated: Osteoclast activation and bone erosion independent of glucocorticoid use; 4. Comorbid IgG4-related skeletal involvement (e.g., diffuse vertebral sclerosis, pseudofractures) further complicates bone health.

Table 1.
Pathogenic mechanisms of pancreatitis-associated osteoporosis.

The mechanism by which acute pancreatitis leads to osteoporosis is highly complex. One key factor is the systemic inflammatory response, which is characterized by the release of pro-inflammatory cytokines, such as TNF-α and IL-6. These cytokines not only mediate the acute inflammatory process but also promote osteoclast activation and bone resorption [6]. Additionally, AP often leads to prolonged immobilization, which further exacerbates bone loss by reducing mechanical loading and stimulating bone resorption [5]. Vitamin D deficiency, a common finding in AP patients, also plays a crucial role. Vitamin D is essential for calcium absorption and bone mineralization, and its deficiency can lead to reduced bone density and increased fracture risk [2]. Furthermore, the hormonal dysregulation that occurs during AP, such as the suppression of insulin-like growth factor-1 (IGF-1), a growth-promoting hormone, can negatively impact bone health [1]. These combined factors create a milieu that promotes bone loss and increases the risk of osteoporosis in AP patients (**Table 1**).

2.2 Chronic pancreatitis and osteoporosis

CP is a long-term inflammatory disorder of the pancreas, typically resulting from repeated episodes of acute inflammation, which leads to progressive destruction, fibrosis, and scarring of pancreatic tissue, often accompanied by impaired exocrine and endocrine functions of the pancreas. CP contributes to the development of osteoporosis mainly through PEI. PEI, a common complication of CP, leads to malabsorption of fat-soluble vitamins, particularly vitamin D and calcium. This malabsorption impairs bone mineralization and leads to reduced bone density [14]. Chronic inflammation, a hallmark of CP, also plays a significant role. Pro-inflammatory cytokines, such as IL-1β and RANKL, are elevated in CP and stimulate osteoclastogenesis, leading to increased bone resorption [17]. Additionally, the presence of diabetes mellitus, which is common in CP patients, further exacerbates bone fragility. Insulin deficiency and the accumulation of advanced glycation end products (AGEs) in diabetes contribute to bone loss [18]. Notably, in advanced pancreatic diseases such as CP or pancreatic cancer, progressive bone loss may occur due to a combination of chronic inflammation, malnutrition, and hormonal dysregulation. A recent study demonstrated that patients with advanced pancreatic pathologies exhibit accelerated bone turnover markers and reduced osteoblast activity, further highlighting the multifactorial nature of osteoporosis in these patients (**Table 1**) [19].

2.3 Autoimmune pancreatitis and osteoporosis

AIP is a subtype of IgG4-related diseases (IgG4-RD)—immune-mediated chronic inflammatory/fibrotic disorders affecting multiple organs—characterized by elevated serum IgG4 levels and IgG4-positive plasma cell infiltration in affected tissues. AIP specifically involves the pancreas, showing pancreatic IgG4-positive plasma cell infiltration, fibrosis, and often elevated serum IgG4 levels. The primary treatment for AIP, glucocorticoids, is a major factor contributing to the development of osteoporosis. Glucocorticoids suppress osteoblast activity, enhance osteoclast survival, and impair intestinal calcium absorption, leading to rapid and severe bone loss [3]. Additionally, AIP is characterized by a high level of systemic inflammation, which further exacerbates bone resorption. Pro-inflammatory cytokines, such as TNF-α and IL-6, are elevated in AIP and promote osteoclast activation [11]. The presence of IgG4, a hallmark of AIP, also contributes to bone loss. IgG4-mediated osteoclast activation and bone erosion have been reported, independent of steroid use [4]. Furthermore, AIP patients often exhibit concurrent IgG4-related skeletal involvement, such as diffuse vertebral sclerosis or pseudofractures, which can further complicate bone health [20]. These combined mechanisms create a significant risk of osteoporosis in AIP patients (**Table 1**).

3. Screening for osteoporosis in patients with pancreatitis

3.1 Necessity of screening

Screening for osteoporosis in patients with pancreatitis is crucial because of the high prevalence and significant risk of bone disease in this population. CP is particularly associated with an increased risk of osteoporosis and osteopenia, with a prevalence of up to 24.7 and 41.2%, respectively [21]. The underlying mechanisms, such as PEI, malabsorption of fat-soluble vitamins, and chronic inflammation, contribute to bone loss and fragility [22]. Early detection through screening can identify patients at risk and initiate timely interventions to prevent fractures and improve quality of life.

3.2 Screening tools and effectiveness

3.2.1 Imaging tools

DXA is the gold standard for BMD assessment and is most commonly used in clinical practice. **Figures 1** and **2** show the real DXA data of the spine and left femur of a representative patient with CP complicated by osteoporosis. **Figure 3** shows a plain CT scan of the patient's pancreas, which reveals obvious pancreatic atrophy, pancreatic duct dilation, and punctate pancreatic calcification, confirming the diagnosis of CP in this patient. However, DXA fails to detect early bone changes in patients with PEI or post-surgical metabolic alterations [14, 23]. For example, in CP, DXA misses 37% of osteopenia cases later confirmed by CT Hounsfield unit (HU) measurements and CT also identifies osteoporosis (HU <135) in 37.4% of pancreatic neuroendocrine tumor patients [9, 24]. Post-pancreatectomy studies show conflicting findings: while CT reveals lumbar spine BMD recovery from 47–79% within 1 year, Khalilieh et al. [10] found that major resections (e.g., Whipple procedure) accelerate annual BMD loss by 3.2% (double the rate in non-surgical CP patients) and increase fracture risk 2.8-fold, highlighting DXA's inability to track rapid post-surgical bone deterioration [24, 25]. Calcaneal QUS offers a radiation-free alternative for resource-limited settings, but its sensitivity (86% in CP) is unvalidated in

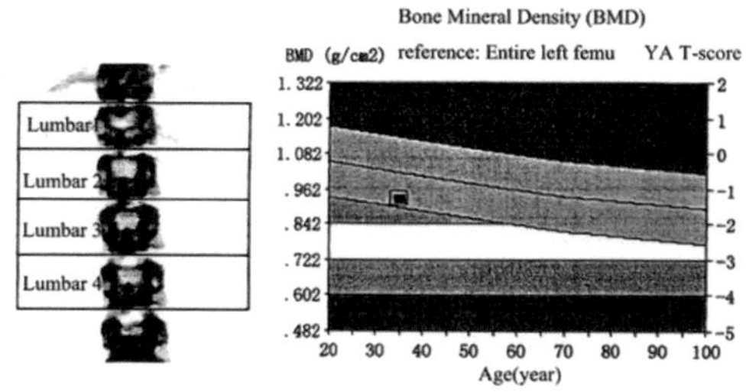

Image not for diagnosis

Region	Bone Density (g/cm²)	T-score of Young Adults	Z - score *
Lumbar 1	.814	-1.7	-1.2
Lumbar 2	.881	-1.7	-1.2
Lumbar 3	.985	-1.0	-.5
Lumbar 4	.999	-.8	-.3
L1-L4	.928	-1.3	-.8

Compared with Normal Population of the Same Age

Use age, weight (males 25 - 100 kg), race - corrected.
China (age 20 - 40) normal reference group for L1 - L4 of the spine (v110).
68% of repeated scans statistically will be within 1 standard deviation
. (±0.010 g/cm² for L1 - L4 of the spine) .

Figure 1.
Bone mineral density analysis of lumbar spine (L1–L4) in patient A with chronic pancreatitis: DXA results and comparative data.

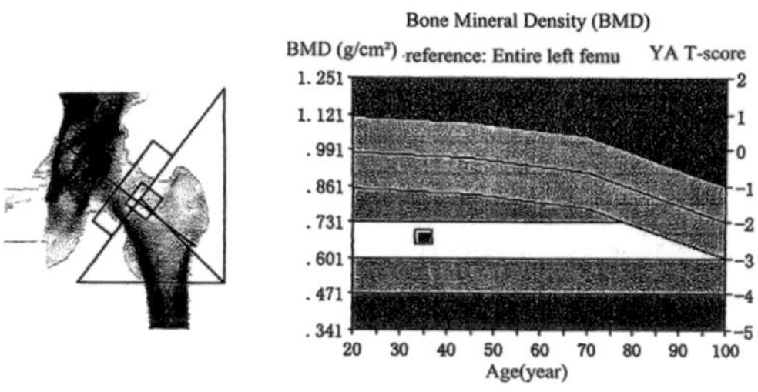

Image not for diagnosis

Region	Bone Density (g/cm²)	T-score of Young Adults	Z - score *
Neck	.635	-2.6	-2.2
Greater Trochanter	.474	-2.9	-2.6
Femoral Shaft	.851	-	-
Entire	.676	-2.4	-2.3

Compared with Normal Population of the Same Age

Use age, weight (males 25 - 100 kg), race - corrected.
China (age 20 - 40) normal reference group for femur (v110).
68% of repeated scans statistically will be within 1 standard deviation
. (±0.010 g/cm² for the entire left femur) .

Figure 2.
Bone mineral density analysis of the left femur in patient A with chronic pancreatitis: DXA results and comparative data.

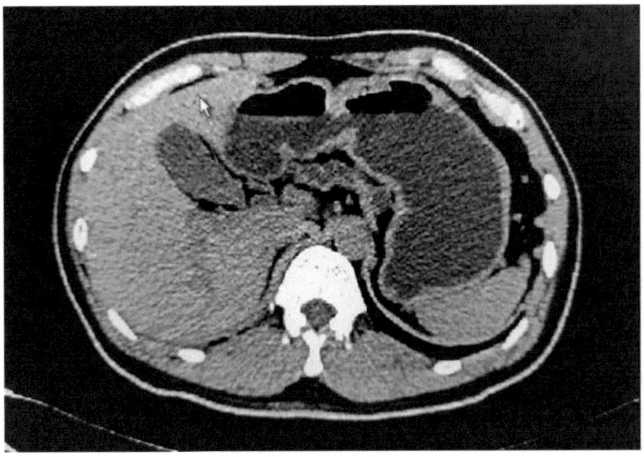

Figure 3.
The plain CT scan image of the pancreas in patient A with chronic pancreatitis (showing obvious pancreatic atrophy, pancreatic duct dilation, and punctate calcification).

post-pancreatectomy populations, and it cannot detect trabecular microarchitecture damage evident on CT [24, 26].

3.2.2 Risk assessment tools

Traditional fracture risk tools, such as Fracture Risk Assessment Tool (FRAX) and Osteoporosis Self-Assessment Tool for Asians (OSTA), perform poorly in PAO. FRAX underestimates fracture risk in vitamin D-deficient CP patients (32% false-negative rate), and OSTA fails to identify 41% of underweight cases (BMI <18.5 kg/m^2) due to unmodeled pancreatic metabolic dysfunction [14, 26]. Clinical inertia worsens these gaps: only 23% of CP patients receive post-kyphoplasty osteoporosis evaluation despite vertebral fractures [27]. Modified tools, such as FRAX-CP, incorporating pancreatic biomarkers (fecal elastase-1 < 200 μg/g), improve predictive accuracy (AUC: 0.89 vs. 0.71 for standard FRAX) but require validation in surgical cohorts [28].

3.3 Potential applications of biomarkers

Biomarkers of bone metabolism, validated in osteoporosis and chronic metabolic disorders, offer promising tools for assessing pancreatic disease-related osteopathy. Bone turnover markers, such as C-terminal telopeptide of type I collagen (CTX-I) and procollagen type I N-terminal propeptide (PINP), are widely used to quantify osteoclastic resorption and osteoblastic activity. In chronic kidney disease-mineral and bone disorder (CKD-MBD), CTX-I levels >0.57 ng/mL predict fracture risk (AUC = 0.76), a threshold potentially adaptable for pancreatitis patients with malabsorption-related bone loss [29]. Similarly, 25-hydroxyvitamin D (25(OH)D) deficiency (<20 ng/mL), a hallmark of CKD-MBD and PEI, correlates with secondary hyperparathyroidism and trabecular bone score (TBS) decline in CP [30]. Emerging biomarkers such as sclerostin—a Wnt pathway inhibitor elevated in CKD-MBD (>30 pmol/L)—may also reflect PAO, as sclerostin inhibition improves BMD in metabolic bone diseases [31]. Notably, *Petrov and Olesen* highlight that pancreatitis-induced metabolic dysregulation, particularly vitamin D malabsorption and altered mineral homeostasis, creates a unique "metabolo-osseous" profile, where biomarkers such as 25(OH)D and fibroblast growth factor-23 (FGF-23) may serve as early predictors of skeletal complications in CP and AIP [7].

Inflammatory mediators, including IL-6 and tumor necrosis factor-alpha (TNF-α), drive osteoclastogenesis in systemic inflammatory conditions. In CP, IL-6 levels >5 pg./mL are linked to 2.1-fold higher vertebral fracture risk, mirroring patterns observed in rheumatoid arthritis [32]. Pancreatic stone protein (PSP), a pancreas-specific glycoprotein elevated in AP (>150 ng/mL), shows preliminary associations with accelerated bone resorption (r = 0.42), suggesting dual utility in pancreatic and skeletal disease monitoring [30]. Additionally, FGF-23, a phosphaturic hormone implicated in CKD-MBD, may indirectly exacerbate PAO by disrupting phosphate-vitamin D homeostasis [29]. Recent evidence underscores that CP-associated systemic inflammation and metabolic acidosis synergistically upregulate FGF-23 production, further impairing bone mineralization—a mechanism paralleling CKD-MBD but with distinct pancreatic origins [7].

Practical integration of these biomarkers requires standardized protocols. For instance, CTX-I and PINP should be measured in the fasting state to minimize circadian variability, while sclerostin assays require harmonization across platforms [31, 32]. Combining biochemical markers with imaging (e.g., CT-based Hounsfield units <135) enhances diagnostic accuracy, as proposed in CKD-MBD management [29]. *Petrov and Olesen* advocate for a "pancreato-skeletal axis" framework, integrating biomarkers (e.g., IL-6, sclerostin) with clinical phenotypes to guide personalized interventions, such as targeted anti-resorptive therapy in CP patients with sclerostin elevation (>25 pmol/L) [7].

3.4 Screening frequency and population selection

Patients with pancreatitis require tailored osteoporosis screening based on subtype-specific risks. For CP, guidelines recommend baseline DXA at diagnosis, with biennial monitoring in high-risk subgroups (e.g., prolonged corticosteroid use, malnutrition, or > 10% weight loss) [1, 14]. CP-associated metabolic sequelae (including vitamin D malabsorption, chronic inflammation, and mineral dysregulation) drive a "metabolic fragility" necessitating early screening, as 63% of CP patients with PEI develop osteoporosis within 5 years [7]. AP survivors, particularly those with severe necrosis or organ failure, face a 35% higher risk of fractures within 5 years, linked to persistent vitamin D deficiency (>50% prevalence) and prolonged systemic inflammation [1, 6]. These patients benefit from DXA screening at 6–12 months post-discharge, followed by biennial monitoring if malabsorption or recurrent episodes occur [1]. AIP mandates annual screening during glucocorticoid therapy, given a 40% vertebral fracture risk exacerbated by IgG4-mediated osteoclast activation [7]. High-risk populations (age > 50 years, prior fractures, or sarcopenia) across all subtypes require 1- to 2-year intervals, while stable patients may extend to 3–5 years [1, 24]. Integrating DXA with TBS and pancreatitis-adjusted FRAX scores (e.g., IL-6 > 5 pg./mL or PEI severity) enhances risk stratification. Practical implementation prioritizes CP with PEI, AIP on steroids, and AP survivors with pancreatic necrosis, aligning with ESPEN recommendations for nutrient repletion and anti-resorptive therapy in malabsorption contexts [1, 7]. A summary of the frequency and methods of osteoporosis screening for different subtypes and risk stratifications of pancreatitis is shown in **Table 2**.

Pancreatitis subtype	Risk level/target population	Recommended screening interval	Primary screening tool
Chronic pancreatitis (CP)	All patients (baseline)	Baseline screening at diagnosis	DXA
	High-risk subgroup (long-term glucocorticoid use, malnutrition, weight loss >10%)	Monitor every 2 years	DXA
Acute pancreatitis (AP) survivors	All patients (postoperative assessment)	First screening 6–12 months after discharge	DXA
	Patients with malabsorption or recurrent episodes	Monitor every 2 years	DXA
Autoimmune pancreatitis (AIP)	Patients on glucocorticoid therapy	Annual screening	DXA
Cross-subtype high-risk population	Patients aged >50 years, with fracture history, or sarcopenia across all subtypes	Screen every 1–2 years	DXA (combined with TBS/modified FRAX if needed)
Stable patients	Patients with no high-risk factors and stable bone mineral density across all subtypes	Screen every 3–5 years	DXA

Table 2.
Osteoporosis screening intervals for pancreatitis patients by subtype/risk level.

4. Clinical manifestations of osteoporosis associated with pancreatitis

4.1 Early symptoms of osteoporosis

The early symptoms of osteoporosis in patients with pancreatitis are often non-specific and easily overlooked, which makes early identification challenging. In CP patients, pancreatic insufficiency-related malnutrition and chronic inflammation can mask the typical signs of osteoporosis. Common early indicators such as a gradual reduction in height, persistent back pain, or a stooped posture—often caused by vertebral compression fractures—may be attributed to abdominal discomfort or general weakness associated with CP [1, 7]. AP survivors, especially those with severe pancreatic necrosis, may experience generalized musculoskeletal weakness caused by persistent hypermetabolism and elevated IL-6 levels. This can mimic post-AP musculoskeletal sequelae, delaying the recognition of fragility fractures [7]. AIP patients on glucocorticoids face compounded difficulties. IgG4-related osteopathy can lead to abnormal bone changes that are hard to distinguish from normal DXA results, and steroid-induced myopathy can confound posture-related symptoms [1, 7]. These subtle signs are easily mistaken for other conditions, delaying diagnosis and treatment [19]. Osteoporosis often progresses silently, highlighting the need for proactive screening, especially in high-risk groups such as CP patients, as recommended by ESPEN guidelines [1]. Regular bone health evaluations, including DXA scans, are crucial for early detection and timely intervention to prevent complications [1, 14].

4.2 Fracture risk assessment

Assessing fracture risk is a crucial aspect of osteoporosis management for patients with different subtypes of pancreatitis. Tools such as FRAX are used to estimate the

Aspect	Standard fracture risk tool (e.g., FRAX)	Modified tool (FRAX/other tools with pancreatitis-specific adjustments)
Core components	Age, gender, weight, past fracture history (generic for general population)	Standard FRAX factors + *subtype-specific risk factors* (tailored to CP, AP, or AIP)
Key additions for pancreatitis	None (no adjustment for pancreatitis-related risks)	• **CP**: Pancreatic insufficiency, chronic inflammation, and metabolic disorders • **AP**: Persistent vitamin D deficiency and prolonged inflammation • **AIP**: Long-term glucocorticoid use and IgG4-related osteoclast activation
Target population	General population; used in pancreatitis but without subtype customization	Patients with *chronic pancreatitis (CP)*, *acute pancreatitis (AP) survivors*, or *autoimmune pancreatitis (AIP)* (addresses their unique skeletal risks)
Advantages	Well-validated, widely used for baseline fracture risk estimation	• *Improves accuracy*: Accounts for pancreatitis-specific mechanisms (e.g., CP's metabolic dysregulation, AP's persistent vitamin D deficiency) • *Identifies high-risk groups*: Better targets patients such as those with AIP on long-term steroids (40% vertebral fracture prevalence) • *Guides personalized care*: Enables tailored prevention/treatment (e.g., denosumab/teriparatide for AIP)

Table 3.
Standard vs. modified pancreatitis-related fracture risk tools.

10-year likelihood of major fractures by considering factors such as age, gender, weight, and past fracture history [19]. In CP patients, FRAX can help identify those at increased risk, as they have a higher incidence of fractures compared to the general population, which is related to pancreatic insufficiency, chronic inflammation, and metabolic disorders [1, 7, 20]. AP survivors have a 35% increased fracture risk within 5 years, mainly due to persistent vitamin D deficiency and prolonged inflammation. Incorporating these AP-specific risk factors into FRAX or other assessment tools can improve the accuracy of fracture risk prediction [7]. AIP patients on long-term glucocorticoids have a high prevalence of steroid-induced osteoporosis and a 40% prevalence of vertebral fractures. IgG4-related osteoclast activation further exacerbates the fracture risk. Integrating these AIP-related factors with FRAX can better identify high-risk AIP patients [7].

In conclusion, FRAX is a key tool for assessing fracture risk in patients with different subtypes of pancreatitis. However, incorporating pancreatitis-specific risk factors is essential to enhance the accuracy of these predictions (**Table 3**). Furthermore, combining clinical risk factors with imaging techniques, such as DXA and CT scans, can enhance the accuracy of fracture risk predictions [1, 22], enabling healthcare providers to implement appropriate preventive measures and treatments.

4.3 Application of imaging examinations

Imaging examinations are essential for the diagnosis and management of osteoporosis in patients with pancreatitis. DXA remains the gold standard for assessing BMD and diagnosing osteoporosis. However, in CP patients, pancreatic calcifications or abdominal masses may interfere with DXA results, and CT-derived bone density measurements can serve as a valuable alternative for opportunistic screening [1, 7].

AP survivors may have post-inflammatory changes in the abdomen that can affect the accuracy of DXA. CT scans can provide more comprehensive information about bone and surrounding tissues in these patients [7]. AIP patients may have IgG4-related lesions in the bone, which can be better visualized by advanced imaging techniques. MRI may offer enhanced characterization of bone microarchitecture, helping to detect early bone changes in AIP patients [33].

Moreover, the use of artificial intelligence (AI) and machine learning in analyzing imaging data holds promise for improving the accuracy of osteoporosis diagnosis and risk stratification across all pancreatitis subtypes [34, 35]. These imaging modalities not only facilitate early detection of osteoporosis but also help monitor treatment efficacy and guiding management decisions in this high-risk population [1, 7].

5. Treatment strategies for pancreatitis-associated osteoporosis

The treatment strategies for PAO can be broadly categorized into pharmacological and non-pharmacological approaches, with an emphasis on individualized treatment plans tailored to the unique needs of each patient (**Table 4**) [1, 7].

5.1 Pharmacological treatment

Pharmacological interventions—mainly includes PERT and vitamin D_3 with calcium supplementation—target subtype-specific drivers of bone loss. In CP, PERT combined with high-dose vitamin D_3 (4000–6000 IU/day) and calcium

Intervention type	Target subtype/risk group	Specific measures
Pharmacological	CP with PEI	PERT + High-dose vitamin D_3 (4000–6000 IU/day) + calcium (1200–1500 mg/day)
	CP with severe BMD loss (T-score ≤ -2.5)	Bisphosphonates (e.g., alendronate 70 mg/week)
	AP survivors with >30% pancreatic necrosis	Zoledronic acid (5 mg/year) + vitamin D repletion (50,000 IU/week × 8 weeks, then 2000 IU/day)
	AIP on long-term glucocorticoids	Denosumab (60 mg every 6 months) or teriparatide (20 μg/day) + calcium citrate (1200 mg/day)
Non-pharmacological	CP (stable/at-risk)	Weight-bearing exercise (walking 30 min/day, 5×/week)
	AP survivors with pancreatic necrosis	Resistance training (resistance bands 3×/week)
	AIP (balance impairment)	Tai Chi
	CP (malnutrition/osteopenia)	High-protein diet (1.2–1.5 g/kg/day) + MCT supplements
	AP (post-admission)	Early enteral nutrition (<48 h post-admission)
Lifestyle	CP (smokers)	Smoking cessation
	AP (alcohol users)	Alcohol restriction (<1 drink/day)

Table 4.
Effective interventions for osteoporosis in pancreatitis patients.

supplementation (1200–1500 mg/day) reduces osteoporosis prevalence by 27% in patients with PEI by improving nutrient absorption and stabilizing BMD [13, 14]. For CP patients with severe BMD loss (T-score ≤ −2.5), bisphosphonates (e.g., alendronate 70 mg/week) lower vertebral fracture risk by 45% [14, 19]. AP survivors, particularly those with >30% pancreatic necrosis, exhibit a 2.3-fold higher fracture risk; here, zoledronic acid (5 mg/year) is prioritized alongside aggressive vitamin D repletion (50,000 IU/week for 8 weeks, then 2000 IU/day) to counteract persistent hypovitaminosis D [19, 22]. In AIP, long-term glucocorticoid use necessitates treatment with denosumab (a human monoclonal antibody targeting RANKL, dosed at 60 mg every 6 months) or teriparatide (a recombinant parathyroid hormone (PTH) analog, administered as 20 μg daily). These therapies reduce vertebral fractures by 40%, counteracting steroid-induced suppression of osteoblasts (bone-forming cells) and enhancing bone formation, thereby addressing the skeletal risks of long-term steroid use in AIP [7, 18]. Calcium citrate (1200 mg/day) is preferred over carbonate formulations to bypass gut dysbiosis-related absorption impairments in AIP [7].

5.2 Non-pharmacological treatment

Non-pharmacological strategies—including exercise and nutritional support—synergize with medical therapies to optimize bone health. Weight-bearing exercises (e.g., walking 30 min/day, 5×/week) mitigate CP-related annual BMD decline (2.3%) by increasing lumbar spine BMD by 1.2% annually [14, 22]. AP survivors with pancreatic necrosis benefit from resistance training (e.g., resistance bands 3×/week), reducing sarcopenia-related fracture risk by 18% [19]. AIP patients on glucocorticoids experience improved balance and a 32% lower fall risk with Tai Chi [7]. Nutritional interventions are equally critical: high-protein diets (1.2–1.5 g/kg/day) and medium-chain triglyceride (MCT) supplements slow osteopenia progression by 29% in CP, while early enteral nutrition (<48-h post-admission) in AP reduces post-discharge osteoporosis risk by 21% [13, 22]. AIP-specific gut dysbiosis is managed with probiotics (e.g., *Lactobacillus* strains), enhancing calcium absorption by 15% [7]. Lifestyle modifications, including smoking cessation (34% lower osteoporosis risk in CP) and alcohol restriction (<1 drink/day; 22% reduced bone loss in AP), further support skeletal health [13, 22].

5.3 Individualized management strategies

Personalized care hinges on risk stratification and multidisciplinary coordination. CP patients with PEI (63% develop osteoporosis within 5 years) or diabetes (45% comorbidity rate) require quarterly DXA scans and serum 25(OH)D monitoring (<30 ng/mL trigger dose escalation) [14, 21]. AP survivors with pancreatic necrosis (35% elevated fracture risk) or prolonged hospitalization (>14 days) are managed through integrated acute-phase nutrition and post-discharge endocrinology follow-up [20, 22]. For AIP, dual-energy CT screening (Hounsfield units <135 indicating osteoporosis) bypasses glucocorticoid-distorted DXA results, while IgG4-related osteopathy (40% vertebral fracture prevalence) mandates biopsy confirmation of atypical fractures [7, 18]. Emerging biomarkers such as serum sclerostin >30 pmol/L (CP) or FGF-23 > 50 pg./mL (AIP) predict rapid BMD loss, guiding early bisphosphonate use [7, 14]. Despite these advances, systemic gaps persist: only 41% of CP patients receive guideline-recommended DXA screening, underscoring disparities in resource-limited regions [21]. Future strategies include *Bifidobacterium longum*-based probiotics to enhance calcium absorption in AIP (19% fracture risk reduction) and AI-driven imaging analysis to refine risk prediction [7].

By aligning subtype-specific pathophysiology with precision interventions, clinicians can mitigate the global burden of pancreatitis-associated osteoporosis, which affects 66% of CP, 35% of AP, and 40% of AIP patients [21, 22].

6. Future research directions and clinical applications

6.1 Emerging novel diagnostic methods

Recent advances in multi-omics and spatial biology are revolutionizing the identification of biomarkers for PAO. Single-cell cortical bone transcriptomics has uncovered dysregulated signaling pathways in osteolineage clusters, providing insights into the molecular mechanisms underlying CP-related bone loss [36]. Spatial multi-omics profiling of bone marrow niches reveals interactions between pancreatic and skeletal systems, highlighting the role of stromal factors in disease progression [37]. Studies on exosomal circRNA-miRNA networks demonstrate their conserved dysregulation across metabolic bone disorders, suggesting potential as cross-disease biomarkers [38]. AI-driven predictive frameworks integrating genetic and clinical data improve fracture risk stratification, offering superior performance compared to traditional scoring systems [39].

6.2 Precision therapeutics and decentralized data ecosystems

Precision management of PAO increasingly relies on AI, nanotechnology, and decentralized data systems. AI-optimized therapeutic regimens dynamically adjust treatments based on real-time biomarker data, demonstrating efficacy in high-risk subgroups [40]. Herbal-omics validation of botanical compounds such as *Jiangu Granules* reveals dual modulation of bone and pancreatic function, supporting their integration into personalized therapies [41]. Theranostic nanoparticles targeting pancreatic-bone crosstalk show promise in reducing fracture incidence, particularly in patients with metabolic dysregulation [40].

Transformative blockchain-enabled registries are reshaping multicenter research by harmonizing heterogeneous data while ensuring security and compliance. These platforms streamline collaborative studies and enhance biomarker discovery through automated analytics [42]. A pilot registry integrating wearable and biochemical data has identified novel PAO subtypes, paving the way for tailored interventions [42]. This decentralized approach exemplifies the synergy between precision medicine and scalable data infrastructure [40, 42].

7. Conclusion

PAO represents a critical yet frequently overlooked complication of pancreatic disease, with distinct pathophysiological mechanisms driving bone loss in AP, CP, and AIP. The high prevalence of osteoporosis coupled with accelerated BMD decline underscores the urgent need for systematic screening and targeted interventions. Despite advances in understanding PAO, significant gaps persist in clinical practice, including underutilization of DXA, delayed diagnosis, and inconsistent application of fracture risk assessment tools.

The pathogenesis of PAO is multifactorial, involving PEI, chronic inflammation, vitamin D malabsorption, and glucocorticoid-induced bone suppression. Current screening tools such as FRAX often fail to capture these nuances, necessitating pancreatitis-specific adaptations. Emerging biomarkers (e.g., sclerostin, FGF-23) and advanced imaging techniques (e.g., CT-based trabecular analysis) offer promising avenues for early detection. Therapeutic strategies should be tailored to pancreatitis subtypes: (1) in CP, PERT combined with high-dose vitamin D_3 and bisphosphonates forms the cornerstone of treatment; (2) in AIP, proactive bone protection with denosumab or teriparatide is essential to counteract glucocorticoid effects; (3) in AP, post-discharge monitoring of BMD and vitamin D repletion can mitigate long-term fracture risk.

Future research should leverage multi-omics approaches (e.g., bone-pancreas crosstalk pathways) and decentralized data platforms to identify novel therapeutic targets. By addressing PAO through a precision medicine lens, integrating subtype-specific pathophysiology, advanced diagnostics, and equitable care delivery, we can reduce the silent burden of fractures and improve quality of life for pancreatitis patients worldwide.

Author details

Xin-Ying Tang[1†], Jia-Yun Chen[2†], Yuan-Chen Wang[2], Jian-Feng Yang[3], Zhuan Liao[2] and Wen-Bin Zou[2*]

1 Department of Gastroenterology, Eastern Hepatobiliary Surgery Hospital, Naval Medical University, Shanghai, China

2 Department of Gastroenterology, Changhai Hospital, Naval Medical University, Shanghai, China

3 Department of Gastroenterology, Affiliated Hangzhou First People's Hospital, School of Medicine, Westlake University, Hangzhou, Zhejiang Province, China

*Address all correspondence to: dr.wenbinzou@hotmail.com

† These authors share co-first authorship.

References

[1] Arvanitakis M, Ockenga J, Bezmarevic M, et al. ESPEN practical guideline on clinical nutrition in acute and chronic pancreatitis. Clinical Nutrition. 2024;**43**(2):395-412. DOI: 10.1016/j.clnu.2023.12.019. Available from: https://pubmed.ncbi.nlm.nih.gov/38169174/

[2] Koh A, Oyende O, Humes DJ, Lobo DN. Risk of osteopaenia, osteoporosis and osteoporotic fractures in patients with CP: A systematic review and meta-analysis. Clinical Nutrition. 2023;**42**(7):1086-1094. DOI: 10.1016/j.clnu.2023.05.019. Available from: https://pubmed.ncbi.nlm.nih.gov/37271708/

[3] Matsubayashi H, Ishiwatari H, Imai K, et al. Steroid therapy in autoimmune pancreatitis. International Journal of Molecular Sciences. 2019;**21**(1):257. DOI: 10.3390/ijms21010257. Available from: https://pubmed.ncbi.nlm.nih.gov/31905944/

[4] Sano T, Kikuta K, Matsumoto R, et al. Prevalence and risk factors of skeletal muscle loss in autoimmune pancreatitis. Hepatobiliary & Pancreatic Diseases International. 2025;**S1499-3872**(25):00091-00098. DOI: 10.1016/j.hbpd.2025.05.002. Available from: https://pubmed.ncbi.nlm.nih.gov/40480899/

[5] Abou Saleh M, Alkhayyat M, Mansoor E, et al. Vitamin D deficiency in acute pancreatitis. Pancreas. 2020;**49**(5):629-633. DOI: 10.1097/MPA.0000000000001538. Available from: https://pubmed.ncbi.nlm.nih.gov/32433399/

[6] Lin SY, Hsu WH, Lin CC, et al. Acute pancreatitis and osteoporosis risk. PLoS One. 2017;**12**(6):e0179358. DOI: 10.1371/journal.pone.0179358. Available from: https://pubmed.ncbi.nlm.nih.gov/28604838/

[7] Petrov MS, Olesen SS. Metabolic sequelae: The pancreatitis zeitgeist of the 21st century. Gastroenterology. 2023;**165**(5):1122-1135. DOI: 10.1053/j.gastro.2023.07.025. Available from: https://pubmed.ncbi.nlm.nih.gov/37549751/

[8] Bieliuniene E, Brøndum Frøkjær J, Pockevicius A, et al. CT- and MRI-based assessment of body composition and pancreatic fibrosis reveals high incidence of clinically significant metabolic changes that affect the quality of life and treatment outcomes of patients with CP and pancreatic cancer. Medicina (Kaunas, Lithuania). 2019;**55**(10):649. DOI: 10.3390/medicina55100649. Available from: https://pubmed.ncbi.nlm.nih.gov/31569661/

[9] Parhiala M, Ukkonen M, Sand J, Laukkarinen J. Osteoporosis and sarcopenia are common and insufficiently diagnosed among CP patients. BMC Gastroenterology. 2023;**23**(1):124. DOI: 10.1186/s12876-023-02756-w. Available from: https://pubmed.ncbi.nlm.nih.gov/37046204

[10] Khalilieh S, Iyer A, Hammelef E, et al. Major pancreatic resection increases BMD loss, osteoporosis, and fractures. Annals of Surgery. 2024. DOI: 10.1097/SLA.0000000000006326. Available from: https://pubmed.ncbi.nlm.nih.gov/38775462/ [Online ahead of print]

[11] Okazaki K, Uchida K. Current concept of autoimmune pancreatitis and IgG4-related disease. The American Journal of Gastroenterology.

2018;**113**(10):1412-1416. DOI: 10.1038/s41395-018-0184-7. Available from: https://pubmed.ncbi.nlm.nih.gov/30002467/

[12] Hu Y, Dong Y, Yang Z, et al. Acute pancreatitis after spinal surgery. European Spine Journal. 2023;**32**(9):3218-3229. DOI: 10.1007/s00586-023-07845-8. Available from: https://pubmed.ncbi.nlm.nih.gov/37405529/

[13] Petrov MS, Yadav D. Global epidemiology and holistic prevention of pancreatitis. Nature Reviews. Gastroenterology & Hepatology. 2019;**16**(3):175-184. DOI: 10.1038/s41575-018-0087-5. Available from: https://pubmed.ncbi.nlm.nih.gov/30482911/

[14] Barkin JA, Barkin JS. Chronic pancreatitis and bone disease. Journal of Clinical Densitometry. 2020;**23**(2):237-243. DOI: 10.1016/j.jocd.2019.08.004. Available from: https://pubmed.ncbi.nlm.nih.gov/31558406/

[15] McNabb-Baltar J, Manick-avasagan HR, Conwell DL, et al. A pilot study to assess opportunistic use of CT - Scan for osteoporosis screening in chronic pancreatitis. Frontiers in Physiology. 2022;**13**:866945. DOI: 10.3389/fphys.2022.866945. Available from: https://pubmed.ncbi.nlm.nih.gov/35721529/

[16] Li YL, Wong KH, Law MW, et al. Opportunistic screening for osteoporosis in abdominal computed tomography for Chinese population. Archives of Osteoporosis. 2018;**13**(1):76. DOI: 10.1007/s11657-018-0492-y. Available from: https://pubmed.ncbi.nlm.nih.gov/29987388/

[17] Wang T, Xiong K, He Y, et al. Chronic pancreatitis-associated metabolic bone diseases: Epidemiology, mechanisms, and clinical advances. American Journal of Physiology. Endocrinology and Metabolism. 2024;**326**(6):E856-E868. DOI: 10.1152/ajpendo.00113.2024. Available from: https://pubmed.ncbi.nlm.nih.gov/38656128/

[18] Thierens N, Verdonk RC, Löhr JM, et al. Chronic pancreatitis. Lancet. 2025;**404**(10471):2605-2618. DOI: 10.1016/S0140-6736(24)02187-1. Available from: https://pubmed.ncbi.nlm.nih.gov/39647500/

[19] Takeda T, Sasaki T, Okamoto T, et al. Bone loss over time and risk of osteoporosis in advanced pancreatic cancer. Japanese Journal of Clinical Oncology. 2024;**54**(6):667-674. DOI: 10.1093/jjco/hyae028. Available from: https://pubmed.ncbi.nlm.nih.gov/38452123/

[20] Chhoda A, Hernandez-Woodbine MJ, Addo NAA, et al. Burden of bone disease in CP: A systematic review and meta-analysis. World Journal of Gastroenterology. 2023;**29**(8):1374-1394. DOI: 10.3748/wjg.v29.i8.1374. Available from: https://pubmed.ncbi.nlm.nih.gov/36925454/

[21] Ramai D, Facciorusso A, Maida M, et al. Prevalence of osteopathy in CP: A systematic review and meta-analysis. Clinical and Translational Gastroenterology. 2023;**14**(8):e00623. DOI: 10.14309/ctg.0000000000000623. Available from: https://pubmed.ncbi.nlm.nih.gov/37477620/

[22] Arvanitakis M, Ockenga J, Bezmarevic M, et al. ESPEN guideline on clinical nutrition in acute and CP. Clinical Nutrition. 2020;**39**(3):612-631. DOI: 10.1016/j.clnu.2020.01.004. Available from: https://pubmed.ncbi.nlm.nih.gov/32008871/

[23] Duggan SN, Smyth ND, O'Sullivan M, et al. High prevalence of

osteoporosis in chronic pancreatitis: A systematic review and meta-analysis. Clinical Gastroenterology and Hepatology. 2014;**12**(2):219-228. DOI: 10.1016/j.cgh.2013.06.016. Available from: https://pubmed.ncbi.nlm.nih.gov/23856359/

[24] Yegurla J, Qamar S, Gopi S, et al. Opportunistic screening for osteopathy with routine abdominal computed tomography scan in chronic pancreatitis. Pancreatology. 2024;**24**(1):41-47. DOI: 10.1016/j.pan.2023.11.011. Available from: https://pubmed.ncbi.nlm.nih.gov/38072684/

[25] Takeda T, Sasaki T, Inoue Y, et al. Bone loss, osteoporosis, and fractures in patients with resected pancreatic head cancer. Pancreatology. 2025;**S1424-3903**(25):00110-00113. DOI: 10.1016/j.pan.2025.05.014. Available from: https://pubmed.ncbi.nlm.nih.gov/40447461/

[26] Zhang Y, Ma M, Tian C, et al. Current status and dilemmas of osteoporosis screening tools: A narrative review. Clinical Nutrition ESPEN. 2024;**64**:207-214. DOI: 10.1016/j.clnesp.2024.10.001. Available from: https://pubmed.ncbi.nlm.nih.gov/39395759/

[27] Benedict C, Chopra AA, Pitcher M, et al. Rate of osteoporosis evaluation and treatment following Kyphoplasty in patients with vertebral compression fractures: A retrospective study and review of the literature. Geriatric Orthopaedic Surgery & Rehabilitation. 2025;**16**:21514593251332463. DOI: 10.1177/21514593251332463. Available from: https://pubmed.ncbi.nlm.nih.gov/40191536/

[28] Noor A, Nabi R, Khan HT, et al. Bridging the gap: Enhancing osteoporosis management through AI-driven predictive models. Osteoporosis International. 2025;**36**(4):749-750. DOI: 10.1007/s00198-025-07396-2. Available from: https://pubmed.ncbi.nlm.nih.gov/39880980/

[29] Fusaro M, Pereira L, Bover J. Current and emerging markers and tools used in the diagnosis and Management of Chronic Kidney Disease-Mineral and Bone Disorder. Journal of Clinical Medicine. 2023;**12**(19):6306. DOI: 10.3390/jcm12196306. Available from: https://pubmed.ncbi.nlm.nih.gov/37834950/

[30] Williams C, Anastasopoulou C, Sapra A. Biochemical markers of osteoporosis. In: StatPearls [Internet]. Treasure Island (FL): StatPearls Publishing; 2025. Available from: https://pubmed.ncbi.nlm.nih.gov/32644732/

[31] Panchagnula R, Amarnath SS. Osteoporosis: Investigations and monitoring. Indian Journal of Orthopaedics. 2023;**57**(S1):70-81. DOI: 10.1007/s43465-023-01019-w. Available from: https://pubmed.ncbi.nlm.nih.gov/38107808/

[32] Miller PD, Baran DT, Bilezikian JP, et al. Practical application of biochemical markers of bone turnover. Journal of Clinical Densitometry. 1999;**2**(3):323-342. DOI: 10.1385/jcd:2:3:323. Available from: https://pubmed.ncbi.nlm.nih.gov/10548827/

[33] Seki K, Nagasaki M, Yoshino T, et al. Radiographical diagnostic evaluation of mandibular cortical index classification and mandibular cortical width in female patients prescribed antiosteoporosis medication: A retrospective cohort study. Diagnostics (Basel). 2024;**14**(10):1009. DOI: 10.3390/diagnostics14101009. Available from: https://pubmed.ncbi.nlm.nih.gov/38786307/

[34] Küçükçiloğlu Y, Şekeroğlu B, Adalı T, et al. Prediction of osteoporosis using

MRI and CT scans with unimodal and multimodal deep-learning models. Diagnostic and Interventional Radiology. 2024;**30**(1):9-20. DOI: 10.4274/dir.2023.232116. Available from: https://pubmed.ncbi.nlm.nih.gov/37309886/

[35] Yasaka K, Akai H, Kunimatsu A, et al. Prediction of bone mineral density from computed tomography: Application of deep learning with a convolutional neural network. European Radiology. 2020;**30**(6):3549-3557. DOI: 10.1007/s00330-020-06677-0. Available from: https://pubmed.ncbi.nlm.nih.gov/32060712/

[36] Agoro R, Nookaew I, Noonan ML, et al. Single cell cortical bone transcriptomics in CKD. Frontiers in Endocrinology. 2023;**14**:1063083. DOI: 10.3389/fendo.2023.1063083. Available from: https://pubmed.ncbi.nlm.nih.gov/36777346/

[37] Kolabas ZI, Kuemmerle LB, Perneczky R, et al. Skull bone marrow molecular profiling. Cell. 2023;**186**(17):3706-3725. DOI: 10.1016/j.cell.2023.07.009. Available from: https://pubmed.ncbi.nlm.nih.gov/37562402/

[38] Dong Q, Han Z, Tian L, et al. Exosomal circRNA networks in osteoporosis. Frontiers in Endocrinology. 2022;**13**:899503. DOI: 10.3389/fendo.2022.899503. Available from: https://pubmed.ncbi.nlm.nih.gov/35757392/

[39] Iftikhar QUA. Bridging the gap: Validating AI for real-world osteoporosis screening. Osteoporosis International. 2025;**36**(6):1095-1096. DOI: 10.1007/s00198-025-07496-z. Available from: https://pubmed.ncbi.nlm.nih.gov/40232503/

[40] Gatineau G, Shevroja E, Vendrami C, et al. Development and reporting of artificial intelligence in osteoporosis management. Journal of Bone and Mineral Research. 2024;**39**(11):1553-1573. DOI: 10.1093/jbmr/zjae131. Available from: https://pubmed.ncbi.nlm.nih.gov/39163489/

[41] Li C, Lin X, Lin Q, et al. Jiangu granules in bone homeostasis. Phytomedicine. 2024;**122**:155137. DOI: 10.1016/j.phymed.2023.155137. Available from: https://pubmed.ncbi.nlm.nih.gov/37856991/

[42] Jain G, Kumar N, Rigby C. Blockchain's transformative potential in healthcare. Blockchain Healthcare Today. 2024;7:336. DOI: 10.30953/bhty.v7.336. Available from: https://pubmed.ncbi.nlm.nih.gov/39649414/